Praise for *The Evolved Mascu*

With his book *The Evolved Masculine*, Dest
the world needs. Compelling storytelling and timely content help us all to evolve our
relationships and sexuality. Reading this book will help you not only to become a being
with more depth, compassion and sexual prowess, but will help you to evolve to the
deepest truth of who you are, without the conditioning and social constructs that have
created the destruction of our relationships and sexual health. Read It!

— **Jaiya**, 4x author and creator of the *Erotic Blueprint Course*™

Destin Gerek is THE most informed and skillful educator of conscious masculinity
today. During a daunting era for the modern man, he fearlessly leads them out of
confusion and into clarity, power, and purpose. His wisdom is the guidance every man
should have if he wants to play a bigger game.

— **Eva Clay**, LCSW, Clinical Sexologist and Founder of the Institute of
Intimacy Arts

Destin has created just what every modern man needs! There is so much confusion
and unclarity of what it takes to be a man of real depth, character and passion. Destin
having worked with 1000's of men has cracked the code of dialing you into the essential
wisdoms, practices and mindset that truly will make your life stand out and excel! *The
Evolved Masculine* takes out all the fluff and serves up exactly what you need to be
sexually powerful, emotionally free and spiritually aligned. Don't just read this...absorb
and implement it fully to watch your personal and professional life soar.

— **Satyen Raja** Founder, WarriorSage Trainings

When I met Destin Gerek, he was the Erotic Rockstar. He pranced into any room he
entered, made a scene, and could easily be found in any crowd with his unique laugh.
From those early moments, I felt his passion, his deep reverence, and his dedication
to the mission to educate men on how to be better friends, lovers, and allies to women.
Since those days, I've watched him evolve into the man he is now. While he's changed
many things from those early days, his dedication has never shifted which is found in
spades in this highly valuable book for men in the 21st century.

— **Robert Kandell**, "The Modern Mantor" Author of *unHIDDEN - A book
for men and those confused by them.*

THE
EVOLVED
MASCULINE

Be the Man the World Needs and the One She Craves

DESTIN GEREK

ARCHETYPAL
PUBLISHING

Publisher: Archetypal Publishing
Copyright © 2019 Destin Gerek
All rights reserved.

For permissions requests, speaking inquiries, and bulk order purchase options, e-mail support@evolvedmasculine.com.

This is a work of nonfiction. Nonetheless, the names, personal characteristics of individuals, and details of events have been changed in order to disguise identities or protect the privacy of those involved. Any resulting resemblance to any businesses, service providers, or persons living or dead is purely coincidental and unintended. Nothing in this work should be read or interpreted as an endorsement, sponsorship, or warranty of any kind regarding any person, business, service, or service provider portrayed. The author of this book does not dispense medical advice or prescribe the use of any technique, either directly or indirectly, as a form of treatment for physical, emotional, or medical problems, without the advice of a physician. The author's intent is only to offer information of a general nature to help you in your quest for emotional, physical, and spiritual well-being. In the event you use any of the information in this book, the author and publisher assume no responsibility for your actions.

ISBN: 978-1-7341441-2-3 (hardcover)
ISBN: 978-1-7341441-0-9 (paperback)
ISBN: 978-1-7341441-1-6 (ebook)

Printed in the United States of America
Website: http://EvolvedMasculine.com
Developmental & content editing by Gillian Pothier
Editing by Jessica Vineyard, www.redletterediting.com
Cover design by Laura Duffy
Cover photo by David Gueringer
Author photo by Akira Chan
Interior layout by Deana Riddle

To my ever-supportive and loving wife, Elie.

I couldn't have done it without you.

愛してる

Contents

Part III: Sexual Self-Mastery

Part IV: Understanding Women and the Feminine

Part V: The Path Continues

Appendix

Introduction

She was raped by her boyfriend on her fifteenth birthday, three months before we met. I was the first person she told. The moment she told me, I was overcome with a wide range of emotions. The strongest: rage. From time to time, images would flash through my mind of throwing this unnamed, faceless boy against the wall and hammering nails into each of his testicles. At sixteen, this experience was more than I was emotionally equipped to handle.

Anjali and I went on to have a multi-year relationship. Her rape trauma was ever-present. As deep and intimate as we were emotionally, it always felt like there was something in the way between us. The trauma also manifested physically: I have distinct memories of sitting on the bathroom floor at two o'clock in the morning, holding her hand while she was on the toilet screaming in pain from near-constant UTIs and bladder infections.

Unconsciously, I began to internalize the idea that men and "maleness" are dangerous, especially men's sexuality. As a result, I cut off the connection to my own masculinity. The pain of my confusion, anger, and helplessness haunted me. From this place, at eighteen years old, I made a choice that would the course of my life: I would devote my life to creating a world in which men wouldn't dream of committing such atrocities.

Fast forward ten years, and at the age of twenty-eight, I was struggling. My tumultuous relationship with my long-term girlfriend at the time was a wreck. On top of that, I still had the strong sense that I was supposed to do something big in the world, and yet I wasn't doing much of anything. I was living at around the poverty line, barely making ends meet, each month afraid I wouldn't be able to pay my very minimal rent. After a while I got the sense that these two things—the powerlessness I felt in my relationship and in my lack of movement toward doing something meaningful in the world—were somehow interconnected.

It was at this time that I came across David Deida's book, *The Way of the Superior Man*. Initially, I was triggered by the things I was reading; his ideas around masculine-feminine dynamics seemed to fly in the face of the feminist education I received at university. The ideas he wrote about seemed so absolute. I had learned that concepts of masculinity and femininity are social constructs. They're not real. We make them up. You can do anything, be any way you feel like.

I had spent the previous ten years railing against any notion of gender, asking myself, *Why must it be "masculine" and "feminine"? Can't we all just be human?* And here Deida was presenting a very particular way of being, which he called the "superior man." Deida presents men and women as inherently distinct from one another and proposes that we treat women and men quite differently, especially within romantic relationships. I had learned to treat men and women the same; we're more alike than we are different.

However, I was at my wits' end—I didn't want to lose my girlfriend, whom I adored. I was desperate and didn't know what else to do, so the next time an argument began between us, I decided to try a technique from the book. Instead of reacting to her anger with my own anger, as I had always done, I caught myself and practiced staying steady—not taking anything she was saying personally, not defending against anything, not trying to prove my point or show how I was right. Instead, I simply let her be angry.

I was amazed at how well it worked. Instead of the usual experience—both of us ricocheting off of each other, getting angrier and angrier, becoming more and more volatile, and feeling like we were just leaving more scars on each other after it was over—it dissipated rather quickly. After our tiff, she came back to me with softness, openness, and love. When I shared with her the passage from the book that had inspired the change in my reaction, she looked at me with a smile and said: "Keep on reading, baby."

And so I did. Despite my hesitancy, it was working. More than anything, though, Deida's book helped open my eyes to just how disconnected I was from my masculinity, and more than that, how utterly afraid I had been of it.

While I didn't agree with everything David Deida put forth, I decided that 2007 was going to be the year that I actively explored my masculinity and what it meant to me to be a man in this world. In this sense, I am incredibly grateful to Deida and this book for acting as a catalyst for what would prove to be a profound journey of transformation.

I needed to make very clear to myself from the start that this exploration was not about me trying to fit into the very box that I had previously shunned, but rather, to break myself free from any boxes. I declared to myself, *Screw what society says. Hell, even screw what David Deida says. I'm almost thirty years old. Let me figure out what being a man means for me.* I set out to answer and live into the questions: What is this thing called masculinity? How do I find the beauty and good in it? What are the qualities and values it has to add to my life? And how do I find my own right relationship with it?

When I made that decision, I had no idea just how powerful and transformative this path would turn out to be. At the time, I thought it was just me. I thought that this was a journey I needed to go on because of my own fucked-up relationship to masculinity. It took me years to realize that though my personal set of experiences were uniquely my own, large numbers of men today grapple with their masculinity and understanding of what it means to be a man, and that the intentionality and intensity with which I was to undertake this metamorphosis would take me from being afraid of other men to becoming a leader of men.

We are living in a time in which notions of masculinity and femininity and the roles of men and women are being questioned and have become more fluid than ever before. In previous generations, the roles for men and women were much more clearly defined. You were given a clear road map, and you were simply supposed to follow it.

This increasingly outdated roadmap, however, has broken down. The rigidity of those roles has felt more and more confining for men and women alike. We have had several generations of women increasing their status and power within our society, breaking out of predefined boxes of who they are supposed to be as women, and demanding their choice to be anything they want to be. These radical changes have become increasingly uncomfortable for us as men. They have forced us to look within, reassess our own outdated programming, and evolve our understanding of masculinity and what it means to be a man.

I began to realize that I had been operating under a strong belief that there was no real difference between men and women other than what society creates. I thought, *Fuck that—I will not live in anyone's box. You will not label me or tell me how I am supposed to be.* Little did I know that I was still imprisoned in a cage of limitations, only a different set of them. Instead of making my feminine attributes wrong and repressing them in order to fit into what I was told a man was supposed to be, I had made my masculine attributes and energies not OK. In defiance of society's expectations of what a man should be, I repressed and rejected my masculine attributes and energies and retreated deeper into my feminine, which somehow seemed safer. At least I could not become the monster that so haunted my fifteen-year-old girlfriend.

During my transformation process, it was clear to me that I wanted to keep all of the positive aspects and qualities of myself that I had gained through exploring my feminine for so long: my connection to my heart, my compassion, my sensitivity, and my attention to beauty and aesthetics. It was important to me that I integrate these qualities in a way that allowed me to continue to explore and develop them even further, while simultaneously, intentionally exploring the qualities of the masculine. I broke all social convention and rules of decorum and gave myself permission to find deeper truths that I couldn't find within the cultural stories of "how things are supposed to work."

I crystallized a new vision of possibility of the man I wanted to be, and then, step by step, consciously created myself into being him. I reinvented myself, inch by inch, both physically and psychologically.

I dreamed up an ego that I called "the Erotic Rockstar," and in doing so entered a powerful seven-year crucible of exponential personal growth through my sexuality. Given the depths of my early wounds around masculine sexuality, and with so many confusing and conflicting messages all around me, I wanted to know how to walk a path through life as a fully expressed sexual man while holding on to my integrity and staying in alignment with my values. *How do I unleash my sexuality without becoming one of "those guys" whom I hold in such disdain? How do I live and express in a way that does not cause harm to any of the women whom I connect with?*

As I dreamed him up, much of this "ideal sexual avatar" had qualities and ways of being that I did not identify as having. That, however, was where the game got interesting. I could either continue to identify with these notions of self that were clearly not working and justify doing so by clinging to the idea of "that's just who I am," or I could try on other ways of being. I chose the latter, and in doing so, I brought the entirety of my life beneath a microscope.

The Toltecs, ancestors of the Mayans and the Aztecs, used the phrase "not-doings" to describe the things that exist outside of our habits, our "doings." The concept of not-doings requires you to do that which you normally do not do. In so doing, your experience and identity cannot help but exponentially expand. Your capacity to encounter different experiences, which leads to a deeper and broader understanding of self, is activated. Ultimately, as I came to believe, we are not the persona we like to think of ourselves as. You are definitely not the one whom you try to project out into the world. You are neither the clothes you wear nor the skin that houses you. Underneath all of that is a core essence, and that essence is not to be confused with those other things that may spring forth from the essence. That core essence, beneath all the perceived identity, persona, and social signaling—that is who you are. This core essence has limitless expression and possibility.

As I stepped more deeply into the identity of the Erotic Rockstar, I let go of the notion of *this is who I am, and this is who I am not.* I let myself try on completely different ways of being, and my life became a laboratory in which to experiment with what actually works and what doesn't. *How do people respond in the real world to different ways of being and interacting?* And, arguably most importantly, *what feels good in my own body?*

Living into the Erotic Rockstar archetype provided both a decadent and a harrowing path of learning that led me to more than two dozen countries around the world, a seemingly endless stream of incredible lovers, and a rather mixed reputation. As people projected their fantasies and ideals onto me as well as their own wounds, I was treated as a god by some and the devil incarnate by others.

My seven-year chapter as the Erotic Rockstar ultimately came to a harsh end so that a new chapter could begin. From its ashes, the Evolved Masculine was born: a new, potent archetype that I envisioned and began to live into, one that brought along all of the hard-won teachings of the Erotic Rockstar, metabolized them, and added new levels of understanding that could come only with the benefit of hindsight.

The Erotic Rockstar was a trailblazing step forward on my evolutionary path. It eventually led me to cultivate and create the more expansive masculine archetype of the Evolved Masculine. The Evolved Masculine could not exist if it wasn't for the Erotic Rockstar. Most of the wisdom I bring forward I learned through lived experience (often the hard way), and much of that was through the real-life laboratory of the Erotic Rockstar.

I am not a perfect embodiment of the Evolved Masculine archetype, as the Evolved Masculine is a dynamic, emergent unfolding of my ever-evolving vision of masculine potential. (I f regularly.) The Evolved Masculine is, however, the North Star that guides my journey. I point my nose in its direction, and I walk. I have fallen down. I have made mistakes. I have gotten lost, but my North Star helps me to reorient myself and find my way once more. Over years of intentionally holding this beacon in my sight, I do get closer and closer. I increasingly embody the qualities of the Evolved Masculine—certainly far more than if I weren't holding this vision in the first place.

As I lived increasingly aligned with the qualities of the Evolved Masculine, I eventually became inspired to create an eponymously named company to support other men to become conscious, evolved versions of themselves. This company, The Evolved Masculine, now serves men globally, teaching them about masculinity, sexuality, and healthier ways of relating to women. The Evolved Masculine, both archetype and company, is meant to provide a modern and aspirational model of masculinity for the twenty-first century.

We have an incredible opportunity at this time in human history, an opportunity to rewrite the codes of masculinity and what it means to be a man. Women are making it abundantly clear that the old ways are not working for them and will no longer be tolerated. OK, so now what?

In recent years, the backlash against toxic masculinity has grown exponentially, but I know from my own journey that we need more than simply examples of men behaving badly and strong, shame-inducing messaging about what not to do. My life before the Erotic Rockstar is an example of the unintended negative consequences created when we primarily focus on the problems associated with men and masculinity. What we need are strong, positive role models of what is right and good about men and masculinity—and yes, this needs to include examples of positive masculine sexual expression.

What if I told you that there are aspects of our programming of what masculinity is "supposed to be" that are causing more harm than good, but masculinity itself is not toxic?

What if I told you that your core masculine essence is important and valuable, that sexuality can be a gift, and that you have incredible value to add to the women in your life?

I want you to know that you have far greater capacity to create who you are in the world than you have been told.

I want you to know that no matter how messy or fucked up your childhood or life experience has been to this point, you still have the ability to create an extraordinary life and to be an extraordinary man.

I want you to know that while the times are changing and there is an increased spotlight on men's behavior and the more toxic expressions of masculinity, that being a man is *good*. There is a lot of beauty and power in being a man. Recreating the world to allow for women and the feminine to flourish doesn't need to be at the expense of men. We can adapt to the ascent of women's power in such a way that we become only more of who we are capable of being as men.

I wrote this book as a man who is primarily attracted to women for other men who are oriented similarly. That said, I know that people of every orientation and gender identity are grappling with their understanding of and relationship to masculinity. *I see you, I honor your path, and I both invite and encourage you to apply the wisdom herein as best relates to your relationships or personal preferences.*

This book was written to help you reorient your worldview and remove your limiting beliefs about masculinity, women, sex, and most importantly, yourself. Some of the ideas may initially seem crazy or "out there" to you on first read, as they may fly in the face of everything you have ever been taught to believe. I am not asking for you to believe anything I write simply because you have read it. I have never worked that way, so I certainly don't expect you to. Be a skeptic but an open-minded skeptic.

If I have learned anything in this life, it is that there is far more going on in this universe than I could possibly understand. With this understanding, I do my best to always allow room for possibility that exists outside of what I already know, and for possibility that exists beyond my current belief systems. The possibility exists that what sits in front of me in this moment has the potential to take my entire worldview and flip it upside down to the point that everything I think I know would no longer be relevant, and I would have to recreate from scratch my understanding of the universe and how it functions. This can be a bit intimidating, but it is also incredibly exciting and, most of all, powerful.

This book is filled with hard-won insights that I wish I would have known as I was maturing as a man. This is the manual I wish I had had. It is filled with stories of the most difficult points in my life, ones I had to go through to gain my understanding about masculinity, sex, women, and being a man. I invite you to walk the path of The Evolved Masculine with me.

In Part I: Self as Creator, we will explore the perspectives and paradigm shifts that I used to radically reinvent myself twice over so that you can use them to do the same. As we walk down this path, you will be challenged to take full responsibility for your life and your ability to wholly re-envision yourself as a man of your own conscious creation.

In Part II: Lessons of the Evolved Masculine, I share stories of my own journey of discovery with the intention of inspiring you with possibility for your own life. These stories highlight some of my biggest mistakes and deepest flaws and vulnerabilities. As uncomfortable as it is, I know it is important to share, as it was only through these experiences that I learned the potent lessons that helped me know what the qualities, values, and principles of the Evolved Masculine are. Each of these qualities and principles I had to learn, often the hard way. I did not embody or understand them until I was confronted by the pain of their absence. Now, although imperfect, these attributes are consciously part of who I am and what I stand for in the world.

In Part III: Sexual Self-Mastery, we will focus on reprogramming how you relate to your body, your sexuality, and your pleasure. You will learn about the Four

Gates of Sexual Self-Mastery and the Four Tools for achieving it. You will learn to connect to your sexual energy as an *energy*. By learning to master that energy, you will experience total choice around ejaculation, feel more pleasure in your body than you have ever known before, and learn to have non-ejaculatory, energetic orgasms and multiple orgasms. You will learn how to channel your sexual energy for greater pleasure. Something in her body relaxes when she no longer has any concern about whether you will come before she is ready or not. This opens both of you to whole new worlds of pleasure, surrender, and orgasmic possibility.

In Part IV: Understanding Women and the Feminine, we will tackle the big questions about women: What does she really want? Why does she do the things she does? You will gain a better understanding of what is going on with women on a larger collective and cultural level, and learn how to better understand the particular woman in your life. You will finally come to understand what it is that women are craving from you, and how to show up so that she feels fully met physically, intellectually, emotionally, sexually, and spiritually. You will learn the inherent value that you have to offer the women in your life, and come to a deeper understanding, acceptance, and healthy integration of the feminine that exists within yourself.

And finally, **Part V: The Path Continues**, discusses where this path has led me, and how you can best integrate the teachings in this book to move forward into the rest of your life as a more whole man more firmly rooted in your own Evolved Masculine.

My intention in writing this book is to invite you to unlearn and even shatter your previously held perceptions of what it means to be a man and to become more full, integrated, and empowered as a result. I will challenge you to let go of everything you think you know about sex, and in so doing, open up to whole new worlds of power and pleasurable possibilities. Additionally, releasing your outdated beliefs about who women are, how they are, and what they want, and looking at them with entirely new eyes, will allow you to have connections and relationships that fulfill you both.

You have the chance to create something entirely new, to examine yourself and the prescribed rules of manhood. Throwing away the old rules opens up incredible freedom in the sense that anything is possible, but along with that freedom comes a responsibility. If you can do or be anything, then you must decide: What do you really want? What is your deepest truth? Who are you really? Who are you choosing to become? And are you willing to step fully into your power and responsibility for creating yourself and your life?

PART 1
SELF AS CREATOR

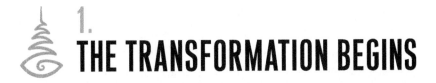

1.
THE TRANSFORMATION BEGINS

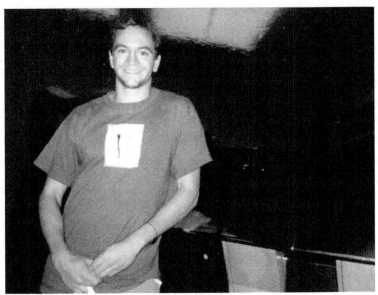

This is Greg. He was a nice guy.

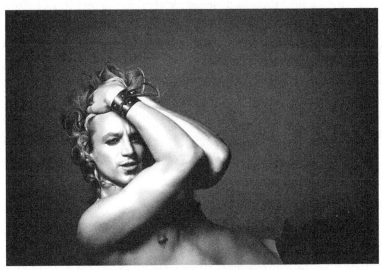

This is Destin Gerek, the Erotic Rockstar.
photo by Paige Craig

At the onset of my change process, I felt compelled to take on a new name. In choosing to change my name, I went for a total transformation of my being. "Gregory" was my old identity, and that identity was disempowered, diminished, and conditioned to play small. In order to release those parts of my identity, I chose to release the name that held so much emotion and old energy tied up in it. The name *Destin Gerek*, translating to "Brave Destiny," served as an anchor to remind me of who I was creating myself to be. Each time I introduced myself and said "Hi, I'm Destin Gerek," it acted as a significant reminder to myself: *That's right, this is who I am now*. My name became an important and powerful anchor for my transformation.

When I first started exploring the ego of the Erotic Rockstar, he was like a character out of a movie whom I had dreamed up and created. I would carefully curate my hairstyle and pick out and try on often outlandish clothing items that stretched my imagination. I would costume up and set out into the night to hit the Burning Man party scene. In these environments, especially in San Francisco, being outrageous and playing with different types of clothing and expression were celebrated, making them safe spaces for me to explore a completely new way of being. It was 2007, the first year of my embodied declaration to explore my masculinity.

Eight months into this active exploration of self, I attended the actual Burning Man event, then a fifty-thousand-person festival in the middle of an empty galactic desert in Nevada. I challenged myself to embody the Erotic Rockstar 24/7 for the full week of the event. I was playing a full-on immersion game. This was a massive watershed experience for me in terms of locking into and becoming this dreamed-up, unleashed version of myself.

And unleash myself I did. Over the course of that week, by day I led eight hands-on/clothes-off sexuality workshops for more than five hundred people total, while my nights were filled with hedonistic, psychedelic-fueled rampages of dance, flirtation, and sexy adventures.

Once back in San Francisco, I decided that instead of simply relegating this Erotic Rockstar persona to living only in the glitzy nightlife, I was going to take him out in broad daylight for something more mundane: grocery shopping at Trader Joe's. I set off around lunchtime, walking down Market Street dressed in full Erotic Rockstar regalia. I will never forget the feeling as I walked out the front door of my apartment: *Game on.*

I stood tall and straight with my head held high. Prior to this coming out, I had made a point of avoiding eye contact with strangers as I walked down the street, unaware of the various forms of unconscious, subservient behavior I had picked up over the years. The Erotic Rockstar didn't succumb to that avoidant tendency. He was not a meek man. He certainly did not move through the world with fear. He stood tall, head held high, intentionally making eye contact with every person he passed: man, woman, young, old, conventionally attractive and considerably not.

I noticed the ways in which different people reacted to this new way I was presenting myself to the world. As I strutted down Market Street, the first thing I noticed was the obvious: the Erotic Rockstar stood out, whereas Greg would energetically hide, and as a result, often feel unnoticed. This was already a major experience for me.

I observed that I had different sets of challenges when it came to making eye contact with men versus holding eye contact with women, but both were a practice of learning to stand securely in my power without shrinking. I had spent most of my life relating to others as if I were "less than," and certainly less powerful than, well, just about everybody. My practice was to neither shrink my power in the presence of another nor to dominate them with my energy. Instead, it was to contain my energy and stand solid and anchored in my own presence.

I was letting go of my old identity as Greg—how he dressed, who he thought of himself as, and how he held himself in the world. I set forth to learn how to do the most ordinary activities as my new identity—Destin Gerek, the Erotic Rockstar—because this new man had to learn how to live in the real world and exist outside of party atmospheres. There's a saying: "How you do one thing is how you do everything." I was bringing my attention into how I did *every little thing*— thus, every banal micro-detail was up for evaluation. The question I constantly asked myself was, "Am I in habit, or am I showing up as I want to be?"

Knowing that I was consciously creating the man I wanted to be, I relentlessly stalked his mannerisms and expressions. I had to answer the question of who the Erotic Rockstar was day to day. How does he walk down the street? How does he interact with men who hold seemingly higher social status than he does? And how is that different from those whom he perceives as lower in social status? How does he interact with women whom he is highly attracted to? And those toward whom he feels no physical attraction? Who is Destin Gerek, the Erotic Rockstar, as he stands in the checkout line buying hair gel, guyliner, and toothpaste? Who is Destin Gerek, the Erotic Rockstar, as he takes the BART train to his favorite coffee shop?

I started to track the moments where I would lose awareness of him. I discovered that it is an incredibly intense process to bring this precise level of presence and detail to every area of one's life—and, of course, it was a long and imperfect process, but ultimately, wildly rewarding.

Inch by inch, step by step, I recreated myself. I recreated myself so fully and so completely that nearly every person I knew before this transformation would say to me, "What happened? It's like you're an entirely different person."

My transformation became complete, however, when I moved away from the Bay Area to Los Angeles. Upon my arrival, nobody knew who I was before— nobody knew Greg. Everybody would meet me as Destin Gerek, the guy who calls himself the Erotic Rockstar. In this literally life-ing process, I learned so much about how people accept you as who you present yourself to be.

As long as I believed I was weak and disempowered, I presented myself to the world as such, and the world believed it and responded to me accordingly. As I developed my identity around being deeply empowered, owning myself completely, and actually being the Erotic Rockstar, the world responded to me as that person: a highly expressed, caring, centered, powerful man who was living an erotically charged, larger-than-life lifestyle.

In other words, how I believed myself to be was how the world viewed me. This created a feedback loop. As I would present myself in a new way, people would respond to me as that identity. Their response would drive this identity more deeply into my system. I could then sink into it even deeper, which led to people feeling it more fully and responding to it from that place, and so it would go.

Through the Erotic Rockstar, I learned the power of working with an almost mythic archetype. Seven years after his creation, the Erotic Rockstar was brought to his knees by heart-wrenching personal loss and family tragedy. Emotionally gutted and enduring yet another intense ego death, I reinvented myself once more, this time as a man who had seen some shit. Not as a man who was deep in the thick of sexual decadence and the emotional rollercoaster of passionate yet destructive relationships, but as a man who had gone on his own unique hero's journey and lived to tell the tale. The Evolved Masculine arose.

If the Erotic Rockstar was about my own liberation, the Evolved Masculine is about being in service to others. As the voice of The Evolved Masculine organization, I have an intense responsibility: people consult me for the wisdom that can come only through hard-earned, lived experience. I created an archetype based on what I imagined the world needed and what I had longed for in my younger years. In the midst of conversations about toxic masculinity and the patriarchy, I felt compelled to create an archetype that wasn't just for me this time but was in service to any and all men seeking an inspiring, positive male role model to aspire to.

With the Evolved Masculine, I learned to keep all of the power and beauty I had discovered about myself and what was possible as the Erotic Rockstar and let go of the qualities and aspects of him that no longer served me and the man I wished to be.

When I initially conceived of the Erotic Rockstar, he seemed far out of the realm of possibility, far away, a dreamed-up fantasy—yet not only did I live into that fantasy, I lived *beyond* what I had imagined in my wildest dreams. I eventually hit a point where I felt done. It was mind-boggling for me to realize that what had once seemed impossible to me as Greg was now getting ever further away in my rear view mirror as my Evolved Masculine was emerging: Erotic Rockstar? Been there, done that.

What had initially been a source of creativity and liberation had come to feel like a cage. I knew it was time to rebirth myself once more. This time, I envisioned myself as an entrepreneur who would build a successful company in service to other men, based on everything I had learned through my journey.

Now, having completely reinvented myself twice over before the age of forty, and having supported many of my clients in their own processes of transformation, I have come to know in my blood that anyone can completely reinvent themselves—even *you*. Your concept of who you are and how you show up and experience the world is malleable. Anything is possible. It does not matter who you are now or where you are starting from.

I get it. As men, we can feel like we are in an emotional vice grip with our entire identity being confronted. Everything we have been taught to be is increasingly not working as the world around us continues to change. We have to make the choice of either clinging to our old versions of self, how things were, and how we think things are supposed to be or else recognize, accept, and embrace this rapidly changing world and commit to evolving, and in so doing not only keep up with but to thrive in this new world.

I first used this process to experience an intense, over-the-top Erotic Rockstar lifestyle, and then I had the tools to reimagine myself once more, creating the archetype of the Evolved Masculine. I needed to shift my identity from a highly promiscuous ladies' man with a party lifestyle to a grounded, committed husband and father, business owner, and leader of men.

Who would you be if you accepted and embraced these changing dynamics between men and women, the changing economy, and the changing roles we are being called on to take? Who would you be as a man who fully embraces the reality of what is and who thrives within it?

You simply need to crystallize the vision of who he is, and then commit—and commit deeply—to walking that path. It will look different from what you now imagine. It will have challenges that you can't yet conceive of, and the path of transformation will bring unfathomable adventure, rich experiences, and fulfillment into your life.

How would your life change if you fully took on the belief that you are the creator of your life? Where might you resist that belief? What becomes possible if you fully take on the idea that you can recreate yourself and your life however you choose, as long as you are willing to truly commit?

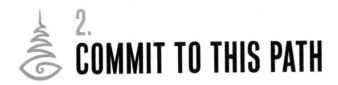

2.
COMMIT TO THIS PATH

This path is not for everyone.

It may not even be for most men—at least, not yet.

Most men seem perfectly content with how things are, even if they are not particularly happy or experiencing the success they really want. It takes a special kind of man to commit time, energy, and resources into bettering himself. You took the first step toward committing to evolve yourself as a man when you bought this book. If you are like most of the men I have worked with, you are dealing with something painful or are struggling with something—and probably have been for a long time—and you have now hit your "enough" point, that point just before the shit hits the fan—or maybe it already has. The way things have been can no longer be. "I've got to do something!" The teachings in this book may hold a key to that something.

I love this point. It is sometimes referred to as a point of crisis. While these thresholds can feel incredibly uncomfortable in the moment, points of crisis are where transformation can occur. As long as you can tolerate how things are in your life, you will continue to experience a barely tolerable life.

You get what you tolerate.

—Mike Ditka

It is when you can no longer tolerate your life as you know it that there is a possibility for change. Change takes energy; quite often, *a lot* of energy. More often than not, it is pain that provides us the energy to fuel rapid growth and transformation.

Are you ready for some rapid growth? I want you to know right now that I believe in you. I have been doing this work long enough to recognize that it isn't an accident that you picked up this book, and since you are reading it, I believe you are ready. And if you are ready, you can do this—whatever "this" ends up being for you. You are stronger and more powerful than whatever it is that is causing you to feel stuck in this moment in time.

Or maybe there is a part of you that is aching and craving for *more*, that sees other men who seem to have it all or who have a certain success or an envious relationship with women or their sexuality, and you think, "I want more! I know there is more to life than this."

Not only is it available, it is available to *you*. I say this very clearly, and I believe it 100 percent. It is going to take work. It's going to take effort. It's going to take commitment.

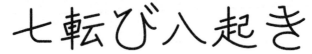

Fall down seven times, get up eight.

In my own journey, I have fallen down many, many times. What has gotten me to where I am is perseverance and tenacity. I know you can do this because I have worked with thousands of men who have done it. I have worked with men who are farther along on their path than you are and men who are not as far along. I have worked with self-made millionaires and broke artists struggling to get by; truck drivers and engineers for Apple; and men from the United States to Australia, Italy to South Africa, Norway to Singapore, United Arab Emirates to Colombia—men from all over the globe who carry the same struggles and desires as you do.

I have seen men who, from the outside, seemed to have it all and still failed to create the transformation they craved, and I have seen men who started with nothing go through this process, successfully recreate their lives, and become the man who, deep in their hearts, they always knew was possible. The big thing that determines whether a man experiences a real transformation or not is rooted in the depth of his commitment.

It's a matter of switching gears, never looking back and be the person today that you've always dreamed you'd be. Entertain every thought, say every word, and make every decision from their point of view. . . . [But since] that person is who you really are . . . just stop being who you aren't.

—**Mike Dooley,** *Notes from the Universe*

If you need the proverbial carrot to entice you, let me just tell you the truth: the number of women in the world who crave and want and need the Evolved Masculine far exceeds the number of men who are truly walking this path. And it is about so much more than women and sex; the *world* is waiting for you to step into your greatness. *Own this.* Commit to the path.

> Have you made the commitment to yourself to do whatever it takes to create the changes you really desire? If not, what would it take for you to do so? What do you imagine will change as a result of making this level of deep commitment?

3.
YOUR BIG WHY

If you choose to create deep and lasting change in your life, it isn't going to be easy. It is going to take a lot of energy, and there will be obstacles, challenges, and resistances that come up. I am not going to blow unicorn smoke up your ass: some of it may be incredibly difficult. What will keep you going in those difficult moments?

Why are you drawn to the Evolved Masculine? Why do you want to create change in your life?

For a lot of people, it is pain.

Have you hit your "enough" point, that point at which something has got to give? You may not know where you are going yet, let alone how to get there, but you do know that the way things are can no longer continue. Something has got to change, and it has to change *now*.

Change can be precipitated by a crisis. After my fiancé, Kirsten, ended our engagement, I was crushed. At thirty years old, I had never loved so deeply nor opened up my soul so much to another human being. I had never poured so much of my energy into trying to make something work only to have it completely fall apart.

Moments like this present a choice point. We can let ourselves be crushed, shut down our hearts, and become cynical and bitter, or we can introspect, explore what our lessons are, and rebuild.

The woman I was in love with was a gorgeous, incredibly fit and flexible trapeze artist circus girl and stripper. She was fawned over by men the moment she walked into a room. I spent most of our relationship feeling inferior. Knowing that she could have just about any man she wanted, I never understood why the hell she was with me. In retrospect, I realize that I recreated myself as the Erotic

Rockstar in an unconscious effort to become the man who was worthy not just of Kirsten but of any woman I chose.

Rather than be that man again, the one who was constantly trying to prove his value to the woman he desired, I used my understanding of women—what I knew of their desires and their secret fantasies—and created myself as a man women would chase after. *If there is an endless parade of women who are interested in me, then no single one can hurt me. If she changes her mind, or decides she isn't that into me anymore, or doesn't like something I'm doing, that's fine. Who's next?*

In retrospect, I can see the defense mechanisms I was rebuilding my life from, and it is no wonder why it was unsustainable, yet it is still a testament to the power of having a strong *why* to drive you forward. At the time, in my mind, the reason my relationship to Kirsten wasn't working was that she needed something from me that I didn't know how to provide. I was determined to figure out how to provide it, and devoted the next seven years of my life to exploring the energetics of relating to women.

Today, I see my big why every time I look into my baby girl's eyes. I see her innocence and her trust, and I am committed to doing everything I can with my life to create a world in which my daughter can feel safe to thrive. Even as I write this book, I am driven by the thought of a young man reading it many years from now, and as a result, shows up as a better man for my daughter. I write so my possible future son can have a guide to help him on his own journey. And I write for you, because I believe that in helping you on your own path of development, I am serving the whole of humanity in its larger evolutionary process.

What is going to be the driving force to give you the energy you need to keep going in the face of adversity and to create transformational change in your life? Get clear on it, and write it down. Really.

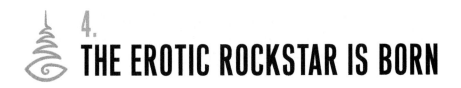

4.
THE EROTIC ROCKSTAR IS BORN

All personality is false. Good personality, bad personality, the personality of a sinner and the personality of a saint — all are false. You can wear a beautiful mask or an ugly mask, it doesn't make any difference. The real thing is your essence.

— Osho

I came across this passage by Osho while living with Kirsten. Every day she would costume up into a different type of character and go out into the world. The world was her stage, and she enjoyed every minute of it.

Between Osho and Kirsten, the realization hit me hard: who I am is far more malleable than I had thought. *If everything I have thought of myself as is really just an elaborate mask that was unconsciously created throughout the years, and, like Kirsten, one can simply change costumes and masks at will, then maybe, just maybe, I don't have to live completely at the effect of my past and the stories I tell myself about who I am and who I get to be.* I started to realize that so much of how we move through the world and who we think of ourselves as are nothing more than habits—a lot of which are bad ones—that we picked up along the way, often in response to an all-too-frequently hostile world.

I have the ability to consciously create who I am going to be in the world?! Whoa. If I can be anything, who am I going to be? How do I break the habit of who I think I am? And who would I be instead?

I allowed myself to take on Kirsten's influence, and I joined her in exploring various characters. I would play dress-up with her and try on different expressions of myself. I would press deep outside of my comfort zone and do things I didn't think I could do. Whenever I would have thoughts such as *Oh, that's not me* or *That's not who I am*, I would challenge myself to think differently. *Well, who would I be if it* was *part of me? Let me explore it. Let me do that which I don't do, and discover what I can be.*

Step by step, I dreamed up the Erotic Rockstar, an ego through whom I could actively explore my sexuality and masculinity. Any and all parts of myself that I had previously held as taboo were now incrementally unleashed. In my identity as Greg, I stood at the edge of the party, whereas Destin was the center. Women felt very comfortable with Greg and easily became his friends, whereas Destin actively turned women on and drew out their animal desire. Greg wore baggy jeans and ill-fitting T-shirts, whereas Destin dressed provocatively, intentionally highlighting his sex appeal.

Kirsten was my muse, my role model, and my catalyst. The circus and stripper influences gave me permission to unlock my sexuality, including my inner exhibitionist and performer. I didn't have much of my own direction at the time. I felt something stirring within me, but I didn't know what it was, and I certainly didn't have the concept of purpose in my awareness. I dove in head first to explore who I could be within this new and exotic world.

In a DJ-worshipping dance culture, the Erotic Rockstar became my performance artist ego. I decided to create my own larger-than-life persona and present him to the world, and people responded. It was sometimes messy, sometimes beautiful.

At first, I wasn't particularly interested in going out on the prowl and fucking a whole bunch of women. I don't think the idea even crossed my mind. Rather, I was enjoying the incredibly exhibitionistic relationship Kirsten and I had— being overtly sexy with each other wherever we were and creating a field of sexiness around us that other people were drawn into.

As our relationship began to fall apart, I bought the provocative book *The Art of Seduction* by Robert Greene. I was under the misguided impression that perhaps the solution was to simply seduce Kirsten back into the beautiful dynamic of love we once had. Sadly (and predictably), it didn't work. Perhaps we were already too far gone by that time. More likely, though, our problems ran deeper than just my lack of seductive prowess. However, when we broke up,

I had free rein to explore the ideas presented in Greene's controversial book.

The Art of Seduction explores a variety of different seducer archetypes. I analyzed which of the archetypes I identified with, and then worked on amplifying those specific characteristics while simultaneously actively testing out and cultivating the characteristics of the other archetypes.

The conundrum about *The Art of Seduction* is that the author is clearly Machiavellian and presents the content without a moral compass. It was clear that I needed to bring my own ethical center to the material. I brought my compassionate heart and commitment to total transparency as I set out into the world, integrating attributes and perspectives from the different seducer archetypes—like the Ideal Lover, the Dandy, the Rake, and the Charmer—into my newly arising Erotic Rockstar persona.

At the time, the internet seduction community (as the pick-up artist industry, or PUA, was referred to) was coming to dominate the landscape of men teaching other men about "being a man," understanding women, and sex. Despite PUA's meteoric rise, it all felt horribly unethical and dehumanizing to me, yet it was the teaching that was most strongly responding to men's desire to feel more empowered around women and sex.

I was adamant that there had to be a better way. This rising cultural force felt like it was part of the very problem I had committed my life to help transform. (While this is a controversial stance, I don't believe that the viral spread of PUA ideology directly preceding the start of the #metoo era is a coincidence.) I became determined to prove to the world (and myself) that it was possible to be highly successful with women and to do so with total honesty, transparency, care, and compassion.

As I became clearer on the details, big and small, of who this archetypal identity of the Erotic Rockstar was, I took him out of the idea realm and began to practice *being* him. It was as if I were in a rapid-growth course in the potency of working with archetypes. Based on the results I was experiencing, especially with women, it quickly became clear that I had discovered something both powerful and highly effective.

Having sexual relationships with multiple women while being completely honest and transparent with them was completely groundbreaking for me. Instead of passively waiting to see what would just happen, I actively expressed my interest in each woman I was attracted to; maintained utter honesty about the fact that I was just out of a relationship, still in love with my ex, and not remotely ready for a relationship; and that I was seeing and engaging sexually with other women, as well, yet despite, or maybe because of, my clear and direct honesty, all five of the women I was seeing happily chose to explore spending time with me.

In some ways, the Erotic Rockstar could be (and occasionally was) looked down on as simply a hedonistic playboy. He had masterful seduction skills, and enticed literally hundreds of women across the far-flung reaches of our planet into his bed. He had psychedelic-fueled, overtly exhibitionistic sex in front of many hundreds of people, and many other high-sensation experiences, like snorting cocaine off a woman's nipples in a Hollywood mansion after being filmed in a music video. A decadent, mysterious boy-toy is certainly one lens through which we can look at the seven-year adventure that was the Erotic Rockstar.

As with all paradoxical examples of intense human expression, however, this one is not black and white. This hedonistic playboy arose out of a fifteen-year crucible of highly immersive lived experience and pedigreed education. It could be said that the Erotic Rockstar came into embryonic being as an eighteen-year-old, sitting on the bathroom floor with Anjali as she screamed in pain.

The Erotic Rockstar began to be built through his rigorous academic studies of sexuality and gender at New York University, which led him to assume positions of support and significant leadership on campus. His passion to better understand the full spectrum of sexuality led him to volunteer at crisis center hotlines, to focus his post-graduate studies on the traumatic impact of circumcision on infant boys, and to be a demonstration model for medical students learning how to perform sexually sensitive exams. His warrior spirit was being forged as a street activist committed to standing up for what he believed in—even when it landed him in jail with two torn rotator cuffs and a herniated cervical disc.

He invested hundreds of hours and many thousands of dollars into sexological bodywork certification, tantra trainings, meditation, trauma education, coaching training, countless personal development workshops and, as a certified daka (male tantric sexual practitioner), laid hands on bodies of every conceivable incarnation. He shared erotic intimacy with women, men, and gendered expressions that exist far outside of the heteronormative binary, treating every interaction as an experiment to deepen his understanding of masculine-feminine dynamics, how different human experiences affect how people are, and how sexual energy works.

The genesis of the Erotic Rockstar was not as straightforward as it may have seemed from the outside. It featured high-voltage pendulum swings, from candlelit BDSM dungeons to the fluorescent lights of the Ivory Tower of academia, and every conceivable place between. He experienced deep, sensual retreats into his feminine, and then came out, with guns ablaze, into big, splashy explorations of his masculine side, from silent meditation retreats to explore egolessness to full-on "everybody look at me!" egoic expressions. It was messy and dramatic (and sometimes traumatic), but it resulted in the creation of an archetypal character so far beyond my own conscious imagination that he became larger than life.

It was from and into this place of devotion, research and development, and obsessive fascination that I immersed myself fully into everything I could find that had something to say about sex, women, and being a man: Robert Greene's books, the ideological canon of feminism, pick-up culture, sociology, kink, strippers, sex work, the porn industry, tantra and other Eastern spiritual traditions, and Burning Man. And at the middle of the intersection of it all, in the eye of a thunderous storm of glitter, condoms, and a relentless desire to make our tragedy-drenched world a better place, the Erotic Rockstar was born.

As you begin to imagine your own Evolved Masculine archetype, what different elements of your environment and life history are influencing the man you aim to become? Can you distinguish the result of external programming from what is your own authentic desire? Are you willing to go ALL IN, and to recognize that there will be mistakes along the way? What might stop you? Are you willing to get this wrong on your way to finding out what is right for you?

5.
CREATING YOUR EVOLVED MASCULINE ARCHETYPE

I first started leading people through a guided visualization process to help discover and connect with their own erotic archetype about twelve years ago. In the time since, I have refined the process by working with literally thousands of people. I now refer to it as your Evolved Masculine archetype—and you can still make him as sexy as you wish. The beautiful thing about playing with this archetype is that he has no limitations. All of your ideas about who you are, who you are not, what you are capable of, and what you are not, don't apply to him; he can be anything.

Truth be told, the work that we are talking about can be massively confronting. It is about a shift in your identity. It is a straight-up ego death. Our beliefs about ourselves—even our limiting beliefs—run very deep. The Evolved Masculine archetype can be anything. He is not limited by your own perceptions. You are literally inventing him. He is a figment of your imagination, so this process of externalizing a persona doesn't confront the ego in the same way.

Your Evolved Masculine archetype doesn't have to be as outlandish and over-the-top as my Erotic Rockstar was. You may find influences from men you already admire and look up to—men you know personally, fictional characters, or people you follow on social media.

Download and listen to this guided visualization I created for you:
http://EvolvedMasculine.com/book/resources

You can find a transcript of the Evolved Masculine Guided Visualization in the appendix.

Let me be straight with you: Stop fucking reading and *go do the visualization process now*. This initial connection to your Evolved Masculine archetype will lay the foundation upon which the key concepts that follow will be built. Seriously, go download the audio, put on headphones, and allow yourself to be guided through the process, now. You can thank me later.

The transformational content that follows will provide tools and perspectives to support you in the process of shifting your identity into alignment with this new vision of your Evolved Masculine self. As you continue reading and are introduced to new ideas and new ways of looking at life, your envisioned archetype will naturally be affected and morph to contain these new understandings.

> Do at least a couple of pages of stream-of-consciousness writing about who your Evolved Masculine archetype is. This will both help sink it deeper into your psyche and act as a reminder as you move forward with this process.

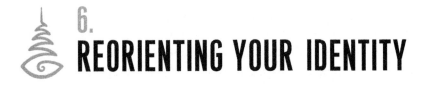

6.
REORIENTING YOUR IDENTITY

What we call human nature in actuality is human habit.

— Jewel Kilcher

We often think of ourselves as static beings. Apathetically, we resign ourselves to thoughts like *This is just who I am*, yet if we are honest with ourselves, we recognize that we are constantly changing. Who you are today is not the same person you were five years ago, let alone ten or fifteen years ago. There is always an opportunity to reinvent yourself.

Science has proven that each cell in our bodies replaces itself every seven years. Every seven years you are literally a new person. Cells are dying and new cells are being created, constantly. Some developmental changes are more obvious because they are aligned with large life milestones, such as when a person moves away for college, starts a new job, gets married or divorced, or has children. Suddenly your entire life changes—and most importantly, you are changed in and by the process.

The truth is, you can change drastically in an instant simply *by choosing to do so, deciding completely, and committing fully.*

By initially crystallizing a vision of my Erotic Rockstar self, and later, my Evolved Masculine self, I began to implant into my unconscious mind, *This is the man I am becoming.* Releasing the tethers of my mind holding me to my past, I decided that I held the power to determine my destiny, nobody else did. As long as I defined myself by my past and old stories about myself, I would forever be in a weakened position.

My past was not something I could change. I could, however, take full ownership and responsibility over each moment, who I showed up as, and the choices I made. Holding the vision of the man I was committed to becoming focused my attention and energies toward moving forward instead of being held by the past. From there, I knew that, in every moment, I had a choice of whether I would behave in accordance with who I had been in the past or who I wanted to become in the future.

I have come to think of this principle as a paradigm shift from a past→ present orientation of self to a present→ future orientation of self. What does this mean? We tell ourselves stories about why we are the way we are, and they usually go something like this: "My parents raised me like X, and I blame them for Y. One time on the playground these kids laughed at me because of Z. The first time I kissed a girl . . . and then in high school . . . my first sexual experience messed me up because . . . and then, and then, and then . . . and that's why I am the way I am." What you're really saying is, "I am my history." The problem with this story is that it is both completely disempowering—and total bullshit.

My focus used to be on the fact that I grew up in a broken home. I was carrying an old story of being weaker and less valuable than other people and that, due to a school sports injury, I was forever relegated to living a life of pain. My identity was wrapped up in my past—especially its crappier parts.

In the cause-and-effect equation, the cause is the past and the effect is the present. The past is the past; you literally cannot go back and change it. The Diagram of Cause and Effect shows that as long as you maintain your identity with the past → present model, you are living your life from a place of disempowerment, solely at the effect of a past you cannot change.

Fuck that.

Diagram of Cause and Effect

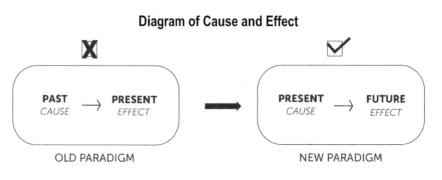

OLD PARADIGM · NEW PARADIGM

By shifting your identity to one based on the present → future model, you take your power back. This is because conscious choice takes place in the present moment. Only and ever. Period.

I took on the belief that *I am who I am choosing to be in this moment and the man I am choosing to become in the world*. Now the cause is in the present moment, and the effect is in the future. I made that internal shift, declaring, "The decisions and actions I am taking in this moment are based on the version of me that I am *consciously choosing* to be in the world." Living from this paradigm of conscious reality creation is powerful.

In the instance of the Erotic Rockstar, I first had to let go of my notions of who Greg was and allow myself to *play in the land of limitless possibilities*, as I tend to say. My inner performer was activated, I dreamed up the Erotic Rockstar, and I began to make every choice from the vantage point of how I imagined he would make it. By doing so, I took him out of existing purely in the idea realm and began to practice *being him* in each moment. As a result, I was creating myself as him.

Seven years later, at the tail end of my Erotic Rockstar era, he was no longer a future vision I was living into; he had become akin to a favorite outfit I had outgrown. Once more, I needed to release my ideas of who I had come to think of myself as. I had to take on the task of imagining who and what could possibly come after the Erotic Rockstar. How on earth do I outdo that?!

I now envisioned a man who could be an admirable husband and father and who could take that spotlight he had placed on himself and turn it outward to deeply serve other men. I focused my attention on the process of *becoming*, and step by step, I cut ties with who I had been.

Human beings are creatures of habit, but we are also creatures of consciousness. Once we do something once, it becomes easier to do it again. The more we repeat a behavior, the easier it gets, until we can basically do it on autopilot. You can drive home at three in the morning while almost falling asleep at the wheel and still make it home. I am certainly not recommending it (though I did it too often myself!), but that is how powerful the unconscious mind is, how built-in habit structures are, and how well the nervous system works. The more we do something, the more the neural pathways associated with that particular behavior or activity develop and strengthen.

Still, we always have the capacity to make a different choice. It takes attention, it takes energy—and it requires that you make a powerful, intentional decision. There is a gap between external stimulus and your habituated response, and in that gap is the powerful opportunity for conscious choice. If you have always done A, in that moment you can choose B. You can always ask yourself, "Is this choice in alignment with the man I want to be in the world?"

Disidentification with the Old Habit Pattern

When creating this level of change in your life, various habit patterns that were part of your old self will have to be confronted and transformed. Start by naming a specific behavior an "old" habit. Doing so will help in the process of disidentifying with the habit and reminding yourself that you are not the habit. Telling yourself "It is *not* me anymore" is crucial. The new habit is who you are. Why? Because you have decided so. As you propel yourself forward toward your Evolved Masculine self, let yourself believe and know that this new habit pattern is more true to who you are and who you are committed to becoming.

You can imagine that in recreating myself as the Erotic Rockstar, I had quite a few habits that I had to confront and transform. For example, I had an old habit of second-guessing myself. That's all it was, an old habit. I decided I was going to take it on and transform it. From the moment I made that decision, it ceased being my habit and became an old habit that I was moving away from.

It is critical that you track where you are focusing your attention and energy. If you are focusing again and again on the old pattern of how you did that thing, then you will stay stuck in the old way of doing things. In the moments when I would notice that I was second-guessing myself, I would remind myself that it was simply an old habit of mine, and then shift my focus toward the pattern I was actively creating and choosing to take on. In this case, I brought my focus, my thoughts, and my words to "I am committed to becoming a man who is decisive and confident in the choices he makes."

When you bring that level of presence and consciousness to your moment-to-moment existence, you become the man you want to be. This is why the foundational step to take on your Evolved Masculine path is to crystallize your vision and understanding of your own Evolved Masculine self and, step by step, bit by bit, *make it real.*

In order to grow and change, you must believe that you have the power to create change. Everything can be transformed, no matter how long it has been a part of you. What would it be like to practice being that ideal man today? What choices could you make to align more directly with this version of self?

You are here because you are ready to do better. Old habits can feel hard to break, but so fucking what? You have done hard things before. In fact, how you show up in the face of adversity is part of your measure as a man.

A year after the release of my first digital offering in 2009, "Orgasmic Mastery: From Premature Ejaculation to Male Multiple Orgasms," I started questioning why some men who did the program would go from self-described "five-pump chumps" to regularly experiencing multiple orgasms (MMOs), while other men made only modest improvements. I conducted some research with my clients, and I came to realize that the difference was *belief.* The men who succeeded believed it was possible, and not just possible in general, but *possible specifically for them.*

Whether you think you can, or you think you can't — you're right.

— Henry Ford

There's a meme in our society that "we just are who we are," and with that belief we define ourselves by our perceived limitations. We have near-limitless capacity, but in order to create change, we must first believe it is possible. You do not need to be permanently defined by the challenges or mistakes of your past. By clarifying your Evolved Masculine self, you can begin ing your behaviors and ways of being today to bring yourself into alignment with how you imagine he would be, and in doing so, take an active role in creating the man you are becoming.

What stories do you tell yourself about who you are that you are willing to let go of? What other aspects and details can you add to your vision of your Evolved Masculine self that will make him so inspiring to you that you will stop at nothing to become him?

7.
THE STRENGTH OF YOUR WORD

The Evolved Masculine is conscious of his words and the power they have. The words you speak are indications of inner beliefs you hold, and they reinforce and recreate your experience of reality. You may want to read that again. It's a big one.

My wife, Elie, calls me a wizard of words. I have now spent many years consciously bringing my attention to my use of words. I choose my words extremely carefully and am in the practice of saying just what I mean and meaning just what I say.

I trained myself to notice when I was using disempowering language patterns such as, "I'm never going to get this right," "I am just the 'struggling artist' type," "I'm not very good at business or with money," and "I am not a writer." Each one of these examples was a story I told myself. Each one reflected an inner belief system of "this is just how I am," and each time I would say or think any of them, I would reinforce that belief in a limited notion of my identity. I realized that this was a form of hypnosis. I was unconsciously convincing myself that these thoughts were truths about me, and I believed them.

Once I began to notice this habit of disempowering language patterns, I trained myself to stop in the moment, back up, and speak aloud what I truly wanted instead. The kicker was that if I couldn't believe what I was saying, then it wouldn't work, as some part of me would scream *bullshit!* I couldn't just tell myself, *I am an amazing dancer who would totally win* Dancing with the Stars*!* However, I could tell myself, *I'm done with being a shitty dancer. It is time for me to learn how to dance*, which led me to actually learn how to dance. I would stop myself short of thinking, *I'm never going to get this right* and instead ask myself, *What do I need to learn to be able to do this right?*

Additionally, whenever I would notice my mind start to fall down a rabbit hole of fear, I would immediately interrupt the "stinking thinking" and re-language the same thought, but in a way that was no longer encoded in fear. In doing so,

I would imprint my mind with a positive new possibility. I would "swipe left" on the fear-encoded version, and do a rewrite in real time in the direction I wanted to grow.

Fuck. This book is going to be a disaster. What if no one likes it? What if people just tear me apart? Or worse, what if it just gets ignored? What if . . . What if . . . What if . . .?

Stop, swipe left. (I would even use a finger of my left hand to swipe an imaginary screen in front of me.) *What if this book helps more men (and women) than I'm even imagining? What if writing it helps me know my work and message better than ever, allowing me to serve my clients even more effectively? What if, by publishing this book, doors open up to me that I can't even imagine from where I am currently standing?*

In the first examples, those words are certainly no more true than the words I choose to replace them with, yet choosing to place my focus in the direction of what I desire helps me move more effectively toward creating what I want.

Words were rarely spoken in early human history, so when they were, they had great power. Today, people constantly talk a lot of nonsense, and words have lost their potency. You can regain the power of your words by strengthening their integrity and bringing great consciousness to each word you choose to speak. It will be all the more impactful because having this type of conscientiousness is so rare in Western culture.

The old magic phrase *abracadabra* essentially translates from Hebrew to "I create that which I speak." When you speak your words out loud, you must know that they are truth. If you don't, then do not speak them. The more awareness you bring to your words, the more they take on a spell-like quality. You are teaching the people around you to know that if you have said it, it is so. Most importantly, you are training your own unconscious self to believe it and act accordingly.

By training yourself to put this level of attention to the words you speak, you can develop a greater awareness of the words you say to yourself in your head, as well. Cultivate an inner voice that supports the man you desire to be, and you will find yourself naturally, easefully moving in the direction of becoming—and being—him.

How conscious are you of the words you use? How supportive or sabotaging are the words you say to yourself in your head? What do you imagine will change in your life when your words are in full alignment with what you want to create?

8.
CREATING AN ENERGETIC SHIFT THROUGH MIRROR WORK

Growing up, my energy was erratic. I was the kid sitting in class who looked like he was on meth, knee rapidly bouncing up and down like it was shaking. My head would dart from side to side, and I would fidget nonstop. I had a ton of energy, but it was scattered all over the place. If I had been born a few years later, I am sure I would have been diagnosed with ADHD and put on pills. I carried on this way of being well into my adulthood. My energy converged around my head, and I spoke in a fast-paced, relatively high-pitched voice.

I came to recognize that everybody has their own unique base energetic signature from which they move through the world. Some people walk around with scowls on their faces. Others default to more depressed states. Still others always wear smiles. While we all have the capacity for any of these expressions and more, we also tend to default to a particular way of being, yet we have the ability to adjust that energetic signature and create a new default state.

I created my own take on what is known as *mirror work* to create a permanent shift in my base energetic state. As I got clearer on the different qualities that my Erotic Rockstar (and later my Evolved Masculine) self held, I would practice embodying those qualities with the help of my own reflection.

Given my erratic nature and my tendency to spin out whenever Kirsten became emotional, the first qualities of the masculine that I focused on setting into my system were *centered* and *grounded*. Being centered means having a calm mind and not being off balance. Being grounded means being rooted in your body, feeling your connection to the earth, and standing solid in yourself. When I was connected to these two qualities, Kirsten could express herself toward me as intensely as she wanted, and it wouldn't destabilize me. In fact, instead, I would have a calming effect on her. Initially I was horrible at it, and then I developed my mirror work practice.

In tantric philosophy, the left side of the body is the more receptive side, while the right side is more active. Through my passionate "field work," I found that when I focused on gazing into a person's left eye, they had an easier time taking in what I was saying and receiving me than when I focused on their right eye.

For my own practice, I would stand quite close to the mirror and gaze into my reflection's left eye (the mirror image of my right eye). Using my eye as a single focal point, I would practice dropping into my body and into my breath. While holding my gaze, I would then let my breathing slow down and deepen.

Using this as a form of meditation, I would allow any thoughts, ideas, and mental chatter to just pass through my mind as I brought my attention back to this gaze with self. I would hold this gaze while practicing shifting my internal state to one that was more centered and grounded, using each exhale as a tool for dropping in. I would maintain the practice until I felt like I had touched into the deepest, most confident, most empowered version of myself.

As I became more adept at this practice, I layered in more qualities that I saw and imagined the Erotic Rockstar aspect of myself to have. As you can imagine, with the Erotic Rockstar, one of the central qualities was an exuded, palpable sex appeal, but there were also other attributes, such as empowerment, solidity, an open heart, and fearlessness. Using a process similar to what I laid out in the guided visualization, I would call him in before me in the mirror and maintain that gaze until I could effectively see him before me, eye to eye.

Initially, it took me quite a bit of time to feel into this kind of energetic shift of my being. However, over time (sometimes with the help of a little drag from a joint), I reduced it down to a single breath: I used my inhalation to call him in before me with clarity and my exhale to ground this new state into my body.

In a social gathering, if I was in conversation (or even not yet in a conversation), there were, of course, times when I noticed I had lost contact with my new energetic set point of the Erotic Rockstar. Either I had shrunk down in some way, wasn't engaged, or was otherwise feeling insecure. When this happened, I would discreetly excuse myself and go to the restroom. Standing silently in front of the mirror, I would intentionally relocate him through eye contact in the mirror.

I would look at myself dressed in my Erotic Rockstar attire and let my physical reflection act as a reminder. In that moment, gazing into my reflection's left eye, I would work with my breath and intentionally reset my energy to source each of these qualities back into my system, finding myself as him once more. No matter what it took, I would not leave until I had him dialed into my being again. Deepening and slowing down my breath was (and still is) a major tool in this process.

Once realigned with this new energetic set point, I would intentionally stay for one more breath, and then walk back out into the world as him. From this new place of alignment, I would reengage. If I noticed that I had popped out again, I would repeat the process until my system could hold the integration. Initially, it took extensive entrainment—and then, like all things, it gradually took less time and repetition. It was nonetheless a process of total devotion— and it fucking worked.

I created a short video to guide you through this mirror work practice. You can find it on my Resources webpage at:

http://EvolvedMasculine.com/book/resources

When you met your Evolved Masculine self in the guided visualization, which three qualities about him most stood out to you? How difficult or easy was it for you locate him in your reflection? What did you notice as you connected to him in this way?

9.
DREAM BIG AND RELENTLESSLY TAKE ACTION

Human beings have this way of creating boxes that we place our identity inside of, and then we believe that we can't get out of the very cage we created. I know I did—and yet, I learned firsthand that it is possible to break out of that self-imposed prison. Not only is it possible to do so in a big way, I believe that creating a grandiose, almost extreme vision for your self and your life makes the jailbreak easier, as it can keep you inspired when it would otherwise be difficult.

By creating these archetypes in my life, first of the Erotic Rockstar and later the Evolved Masculine, I created a vision of self that was so extraordinary and so inspiring that it created a distinctive *pull* energy. It wasn't something I had to struggle toward; rather, it naturally drew me and magnetized my then-current version of self toward it. It lit me up and kept me going, because *YES, this is who I want to be in the world*. Both the Erotic Rockstar and the Evolved Masculine had palpable magnetism—to other people, yes, but most importantly, to myself.

Why was I able to make such a dramatic transformation in my life when so many others fail to change even minor habits? In simple terms, I became necessarily obsessed with the framework for change that I describe throughout this section. I used the principles laid out here to purposefully evolve myself from a geeky but well-intentioned chump to the sort of man who had a woman waiting for him in every port.

I still use these same principles in my daily life as I honor my commitment to be the best husband and father I can possibly be. You can use the vision of your Evolved Masculine self you are creating to relentlessly move toward it, moment by moment, inch by inch.

A Simple Framework for Change

I am sharing with you a straightforward, reproduceable system that, when adhered to, indiscriminately results in change. It is quite simple, but it is by no means easy. For example, every year millions of people around the world make New Year's resolutions, commitments to changes that they say they are going to make with the new year. Midway through January, however, most of those resolutions have been discarded. The resolutions are typically very simple, such as going to the gym three times per week. But they are not *easy enough* to create compliance. This is where your hunger for your own potentiation has to be bigger, badder, and louder than your desire for comfort, predictability, and ease.

Some people are willing to take on changing a habit only if it is convenient. If I don't have too much work to do, I have gotten enough sleep, my house is clean, and I have worked out, then I can take on something new. Until then, however, I am just not up for it. The problem is that by choosing to *not* change, you are making a choice, and it is certainly not the most empowering one. Also, your willingness to do it as long as it doesn't get too hard doesn't consider the exponential cost of keeping things the way they are.

It is complacency that says *I'm comfortable with the way things aren't working.* Think long term. Do you truly want to live your life this way? If you don't, then commit to greater self-actualization, self-mastery, and life mastery.

With a powerful choice comes the idea that you will do whatever it takes. You have to tell yourself, *This is a change I'm making, whatever it takes, however long.* Under this paradigm, there is no "too hard"; there is only *all in.* Recognize that upleveling yourself in any area—even the smallest—contributes to the upleveling of your entire life, which makes the next change easier, and the change after that even easier still.

The following are the simple steps to take to create powerful change to your life:

1. You become aware of the habit.

2. You decide to consciously create a new and specific habit pattern.

3. You notice your old habit pattern after the fact and recommit to the new pattern.

4. You catch yourself in the middle of the old pattern and switch to the new.

5. You catch yourself right before you fall into the old pattern and consciously change to the new.

6. You just do the new pattern, as you have completely integrated it into your life.

Transformation can occur in the blink of an eye, and real integration can be slow by contrast. It is a multistep process. Stopping at any one of these steps is often rooted in lack of self-compassion or lack of belief in self-efficacy. Lack of belief in one's ability to create changes and to have an impact sabotages most people.

As you place your life under the proverbial microscope and select the first habit you want to change, don't just focus on what you are moving away from, focus on what you are specifically *moving toward*. For example, instead of focusing on not living in your head so much, focus on becoming more grounded and embodied. This gives you something to bring your energy toward, which is essentially the new habit pattern you are building.

Miracles are something that the logical, rational mind cannot explain. They often seem as if they come in through means beyond our own. What if a miracle could occur as the result of this new framework? What if you could play in the land of infinite possibilities, and you knew anything was possible, and you could be any way you wanted to be? What would that be like? Who would you be? After all, this is not the time to settle into an uncomfortably comfortable mediocrity, it is the time to believe in infinite possibilities. It is the time to remember you are constantly at choice and that transformation is always possible. No matter who you are or where you are at, if you are ready, you can make change happen.

How BIG are you willing to let yourself dream? How willing are you to believe in your vision? Are you willing to be relentlessly tenacious in your commitment to bringing that vision to life? What is the first old habit you are committing to transform and force into extinction? What specific habit will you develop to replace it?

10.
EVERYONE IS AN ARTIST

I was twenty-four years old the first time I went to Burning Man in 2002. I was in awe of all these creative artists around me. It was very much *they. After all*, I thought, *I am not a painter, I'm not a sculptor, I don't make music. I'm not an artist.* Over time I began to see that my life is my art. The Erotic Rockstar was arguably 24/7 performance art. I created a character and committed to him obsessively. When I was in that liminal space of not quite being Greg anymore but not yet fully being Destin Gerek, I was using the phrase "Erotic Rockstar" to guide my life. I would ask myself, *How can I take this moment and make it more erotic, more sexy, more seductive? How do I take this moment and bring more "rockstar" to it? More larger-than-life experience, more playing full out, more full expression, turning that dial up to 11?*

I dreamed him into being, from the littlest choices he made to the biggest. Not so tongue-in-cheek, I would ask myself, *WWERSD? What would the Erotic Rockstar do?* I took that level of attention and stalked every detail of my life.

I remember one time early on in my Erotic Rockstar chapter, I came home from a party at two in the morning by myself. As I started to take off my belt, I stopped myself in mid-unbuckling-air, and I rebuckled it. I then very intentionally asked myself, *How could I take off my belt more like the Erotic Rockstar?* I brought my hand to the buckle, and though nobody else was there, I completely redid the process as if I were stripping for an imaginary lover or an audience. I dipped my fingers around the belt and bent it down, exposing just a little bit more of my hip below the waist. I bit my lip, hooked my middle finger in the loop of the buckle, and ever so slowly, sensually even, allowed the length of the leather belt to glide out from the buckle, my imagined lover needing to watch with slow anticipation as I pulled the length of the belt through the buckle, let the end slip through each of my pant loops one by one, and finally tossed it to the side of the room in sultry slo-mo, like a male stripper just revving up the start of his act.

Just months later I found myself reenacting this same scene, only this time performing as the only man in a roomful of a dozen young dakinis (female tantric sexual practitioners) celebrating the matriarch of the group's birthday. Little did I know when I was standing solo in my own bedroom that I was in fact (un)dress-rehearsing for a captivating, sexy scene in front of a live audience. It was the beginning of the very public exploration and expression of my erotic nature, which would prove to play a central role in the next seven years of my life.

Every thought you think, every word you speak, every action you take is another brushstroke on the masterpiece of your life.

— Destin Gerek

Everything you do, from the largest actions to the smallest and most mundane details, creates your life. Your identity doesn't need to simply be wrapped up in your past; you get to choose who you are by the choices you are making in this moment and by the man you are choosing to become.

Do you consider yourself an artist? If not, what if you started to? As you own yourself as a creative being, who are you creating yourself to be? What little details of your masterpiece are you going to paint today?

11.
WHAT ARE YOU PRACTICING?

Watch your thoughts, they become words; watch your words, they become actions; watch your actions, they become habits; watch your habits, they become character; watch your character, for it becomes your destiny.

— Frank Outlaw

Your Evolved Masculine self is the version of you that is no longer trying to act out cultural scripts of masculinity that were handed to you by other people—whether family, friends, religion, or the media—but rather, by the vision that you get to consciously create yourself.

> If you haven't done the guided visualization yet, stop and do so now:
> http://www.evolvedmasculine.com/book/resources

Once he is created, you have the opportunity to start practicing being him. The vision holds little value as long as it remains just an idea; the real value comes in taking him out of the idea realm and beginning to embody him in your day-to-day life—starting now.

Remember that Burning Man I went to in the first year of my Erotic Rockstar exploration? I had spent the previous eight months dabbling in the Erotic Rockstar, and this was going to be my test of committing to being him 100 percent for the entire week's event, but it wasn't 100 percent smooth. I remember that first Monday night, decking myself out full on in Erotic Rockstar attire, excited to explore as my new avatar. I hit the playa (what "burners" call the Nevadan desert where this temporary city pops up) with a new friend I was camping with. He said to me, "I've been going by the playa name of 'Pulse,' but this year I think I'll call myself 'Mirror.'"

We were walking across the wide-open desert as I excitedly shared with him about my first workshops earlier that day. At one point, Mirror turned to me and said, "You know, you don't really seem like an 'Erotic Rockstar.'" It immediately hit me like a gut punch. He was right. I had popped out of being him and reverted back to my old energetic patterns. I was being hyper in my expression, ungrounded, and actively seeking his approval and validation of how great I did with my first day of workshops.

"Give me a moment," I said. I stopped walking, planted my feet firmly on the ground shoulder-width apart, and closed my eyes. I took my attention away from the frenzied LED-lit city in the desert around me and focused inward. I intentionally slowed down and deepened my breathing, dropping my awareness out from my head and down into my body. It felt like the weight of gravity increased just a bit, and instead of being on the verge of floating away, I was suddenly rooted into the earth below me. From that newly grounded state, I was able to remember myself as this archetypal version of me whom I had already put so much time and energy into envisioning. I experienced an energetic realignment of my identity as I once more declared and owned my sovereignty, my sexiness, my confidence, and my power. I opened my eyes just a minute later and turned back toward Mirror. I hadn't even opened my mouth to speak when Mirror whispered "Wow!" already able to sense the profound shift in my being.

Anchored once more into my Erotic Rockstar version of self, I asked Mirror to call me out on it anytime he saw me slip back out of my new identity and into my old habits. With that, Mirror was living up to his name. As the wild adventures unfolded throughout that week, I needed fewer reminders. I was committed to the practice of being this utterly transformed version of me. Each time I had an experience that would have been unfathomable to Greg, I believed even more that I was Destin Gerek, the Erotic Rockstar. The more I believed it, the more I behaved as I imagined he would, and the more I created new, sexy, over-the-top encounters.

Every day and every choice is an opportunity to practice. With each choice you make in alignment with your Evolved Masculine self, you further reinforce this new identity deeper into your system, making it easier to access and show up as him moving forward.

You have the opportunity and responsibility to break millennia of programming of who you are "supposed to be" as a man. As you continue reading, your vision of him will likely get more detailed. The clearer you get on who he is, the easier it will be to notice when you are practicing being him and when you are busy practicing being someone you are really not.

In this section, I have laid out for you the foundational tools that I used to completely recreate myself and my expression in the world—twice. If all you do is read through it and move on to the next section, the impact is going to be limited. However, if you choose to, you can practice working with the tools from this section each day, moment by moment, and recreate how you experience yourself, how you respond to the world around you, and with that, how the world responds to you.

Everything is practice, and you are always in practice. The question is, what are you practicing? What version of yourself are you practicing being? Every single thing you think, say, and do is a building block in creating the man you are becoming. This is true whether you are aware of it or not, so make it a conscious act. You will likely find that how you imagine your Evolved Masculine self will shift and take on new clarity as you make your way through the rest of these teachings. Continue to crystallize the vision of the man you are choosing to become, and make every moment an opportunity to intentionally choose being him. By making little steps in his direction each day, you will come to the point at which he is no longer an idea somewhere out in an unreachable future but simply who you have become. At this point, it will be time to create a new vision once more.

> What are the ways that you "perform" your masculinity? In what ways have you learned to put on a façade of what you think you're supposed to be like as a man? What parts of your programming are habits that the man you wish to be would carry forth? Which would he discard? For those discarded, what ways of being would he take on in their stead?

PART 2
LESSONS OF THE EVOLVED MASCULINE

12.
POWERFUL VULNERABILITY

Walking the path of the Evolved Masculine is not for the faint of heart. The truth is, I had no idea what I was getting myself into when I made that declaration to actively explore my masculinity and what it meant to me to be a man.

The following stories chronicle the hard-won lessons and initiations I had to learn on my own Evolved Masculine path. They aren't all pretty. I made countless mistakes. I struggled with finding role models for healthy masculinity that spoke to me, so I set out to become the role model I wish I had had. This is a mighty bold move coming from a guy who wasn't comfortable even using the word *man* to describe himself until his late twenties.

Generally, when I did find men who were older than me and had something I admired, as I got to know them more, I would invariably come to discover aspects of their character that disappointed me. Maybe it was their own hypocrisy, discomfort with their own flaws, and need to present an invulnerable façade, or maybe it was my immature desire to believe in the perfect nature of my heroes. Since then, I too, have gotten a taste of what it is like to be glorified by others, and I have seen enough examples of how society likes to tear down the very people they first idolize. So here I intentionally take myself off of any pedestal and lay it all out for you: the good, the bad, and the ugly.

Writing this book has challenged me in ways beyond what I could ever have expected and showed me more about who I am than I could ever have imagined. In service to the writing of this book, I excavated the depths of my soul to source these stories from different pivotal points in my life. I held nothing back.

I think that for men in particular, the word *vulnerability* has a bad rap. The fear is that if I am vulnerable, then it means I am weak and am opening myself up to be attacked, taken advantage of, or destroyed. Brené Brown has done an incredible job of popularizing the notion that vulnerability can be a strength.

In my own work, I have come to use the phrase "powerful vulnerability." There are two important meanings held in this concept: 1) Exposing yourself to the world requires a certain internal strength and power, and complete awareness that you may experience the full range of responses, from adulation to daggers. There is great power in the willingness to stand exposed and unarmored in this way. 2) Powerful vulnerability contains an extraordinary power within it. When a man has the courage to expose and share the aspects of himself that most people choose to hide, his act of bravery often has a powerful impact and effect.

I am a teacher, a speaker, and a successful men's coach. I could have easily written this book from the vantage point of a man who seems to have it all figured out. Without my willingness to be vulnerable, though, you wouldn't know anything about me or my history, and certainly not my flaws and mistakes. I would have shown you only my strength, the knowledge I have acquired, and the positive outcomes of my experiences. *Here I am, the expert you should listen to.*

I made a different choice because I believe we learn best via example, and I want to demonstrate that the flaws and mistakes of your history do not need to define your entire life. I want to show you that even someone who has faced as much confusion around his masculinity as I have can find a solid, potent relationship to that masculinity—and therefore, so can you. I want to show you that the understandings I have to share with you weren't things I was born with, nor did they come naturally. They were hard-won and largely learned through getting it horribly wrong first, with my pain driving me to seek a better way. When I say I believe that transformation is always possible, my own fucked-up, beautiful path is the reason I believe it is possible for you.

I chose to use my life as an example of one man's evolution, including the places along the way where I didn't do it "right." Imagining this book in the hands of who knows how many men (and women) is, I will admit, terrifying at times. I can only expect a wide range of responses to my vulnerable sharing here, and I choose to do so regardless, because I believe that this is how this information will have its greatest impact on you—not by placing myself on a pedestal as *a man who has it all figured out, and if you would just be perfect like me, then you could have that flawless Instagrammable life.* Rather, as an imperfect man who has walked an unusual, imperfect path.

I have had each of the lessons I bring forward here reflected back to me through the men who have worked with me as clients. As I supported these men through the very challenges that I, too, had to confront, I saw that I am not alone in these struggles or the need to learn these particular lessons. Each of the lessons has had a fundamental impact on my path, and I trust that by reflecting on them, they will have an effect on you, as well. Whether these stories confront you or inspire you, they are intended to be bold reminders of the qualities of the Evolved Masculine that our culture so deeply needs today.

> What are some examples of powerful vulnerability that you have seen in your own life? Confronting the places in yourself that need to change is undeniably a powerfully vulnerable process. Are you willing to be powerfully vulnerable to become the man you know you are meant to be?

13.
CONFRONT THE WOUNDS AROUND YOUR MASCULINITY AND DISTRUST OF OTHER MEN

I had a more challenging time connecting to my masculinity than most men do. Truth be told, I think this is why I am so good at supporting other men to develop the most authentic and empowered expression of their own masculinity. I was picked on quite a bit in grade school, likely from my low self-esteem, which stemmed from my dysfunctional family life. (Or maybe it was that I was smart, wore glasses, and was small and scrawny.) Even as a young boy, I felt threatened by other males. I was often bullied in school, only to come home afraid of what mood my dad would be in when he came home from work.

Anjali's rape deeply compounded my confusion and intense mistrust of men. I increasingly internalized the message that men are dangerous and are certainly not to be trusted. I came to believe that men are a threat to me and the women I care about. What is the impact of these messages on a boy becoming a man? If men aren't safe, what does that make me? I often found myself thinking, *If that's what it means to be a man, then I don't want anything to do with it.*

Without realizing I was doing so, I retreated further into my feminine side. I started spending more and more time with women and less time with other men. It got to a point where all of my friends were women, my romantic partners were women, my roommates were women, and my boss was a woman. I increasingly came to relate to men as "other" and distinct from me. I took on the message that men are the problem with the world and that masculinity is inherently dangerous. I became "one of the girls." Women in my life trusted me. I didn't necessarily turn them on, but they felt very comfortable with me, often letting me into what were otherwise women-only spaces. It was very common for me to be the only man in a group of women.

I was even encouraged to just embrace the fact that I was a feminine man. "It's just who you are." I believed it, and I did embrace it. I found a lot of joy and beauty in being a more feminine man. It led me to having a much deeper understanding of women than most men ever have. It helped me to understand their world in a way that now makes it easy for me to help other men understand women and what is going on for them. It helps me teach men to attune to what women truly want and need, what they are really thinking, and why women do the things they do.

It wasn't until I was twenty-eight that I finally started to realize that something was really off. In my desire to not be boxed in to what I am "supposed to be" as a man, I instead created a different box for myself, because there were all these things about being a man that I wasn't supposed to be.

Simply put, my life wasn't working. Kirsten made it clear that she wanted me to step more into my masculine. She didn't really ask for it or encourage me to do so—she demanded it! I would have done anything for her, but I didn't understand how to make her happy. I didn't even understand what stepping into one's masculinity meant, nor did I understand why. What does how *I* show up have to do with who *she* gets to be? I didn't yet understand polarity.

The difficulty I had embodying my masculine led her to feel like she had to embody more of hers—and she didn't want to; she enjoyed being in her feminine. She pushed me further into my masculine, polarizing me, but I didn't know how to do it. She was upset a lot, and often angry about things that I didn't understand. What was she needing from me that I wasn't able to give her? After I came across Deida's book, *The Way of the Superior Man*, I gave myself permission to actively explore my masculinity, something I had not given myself permission to do before. In fact, I had expressly forbade myself to do it.

You must do an inventory of where you have internalized the narratives that keep your masculinity in a cage of shame or fear. I recognize that there are plenty of men who are still causing problems in the name of masculinity and that this old-paradigm, toxic cultural programming must be confronted, but in order to heal and be your most empowered self, you must address your own mistrust of men, maleness, and masculinity.

What wounds do you carry around your masculinity? In what ways do you distrust other men? What would change in your life by confronting and healing your own masculine wounds? What do you imagine could open up in your life if you gave yourself permission to actively and intentionally explore your masculinity?

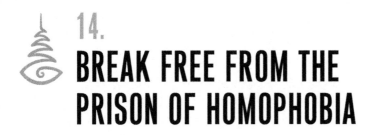

14.
BREAK FREE FROM THE PRISON OF HOMOPHOBIA

I was nineteen years old and recently out of my two-and-a-half-year relationship with Anjali. My heart was still heavy, and I hadn't yet even begun finding my way toward what "being a man" meant. The truth was that despite being in college and on my own, I was still very much a boy.

One day I received a call from Seth, an old friend of my parents, whom I hadn't heard from in years. He invited me to come to Connecticut to meet him and said he would take me skydiving. I didn't know him very well outside of family gatherings growing up, but I was experiencing a real low in my life. I was a recent transplant to New York City without many friends, and I mean, come on, skydiving? I leap for new experiences. I'm there! I said yes to the invitation and headed up with him. I had a blast experiencing the adrenaline rush of jumping out of an airplane for the first time and feeling the wind rush against my face as I plummeted toward the ground at 125 miles per hour. The mixture of fear and exhilaration was quite a way to bond with a man I had always looked up to.

A few weeks later we went up to jump again, only this time was different. That evening, after two glorious skydives and my first official training jumps, we went back to Seth's place. He handed me a beer as we played video games in the living room. One beer became two, two became three, three became four . . . and all the while, we were smoking a joint. I had had very little experience with alcohol and weed prior to this, and quickly became extremely disoriented.

The next thing I remember, we were in his bed, and his hands were all over me. I didn't really know what was happening. I had never touched a man before, nor had I ever considered it. Hell, my experiences with *women* were relatively limited at this point in my life. Suddenly this man, roughly my parents' age, whom I had known since I was a little kid, was kissing me and touching me while I was intoxicated out of my mind, stumbling, and unable to see straight.

What was even more confusing was that as he groped me, parts of it were feeling good. That was even more of a head fuck for me. *OK, I guess this is what's happening now.* At some points, I was simply going along with it, and there were other points at which I contracted, as I knew that this wasn't something I wanted to be doing. It didn't feel horrible, but it was unlike any experience I had had before that had come from my own internal desire and choosing. This felt more like something that was happening *to* me.

It was confusing because we had been forming a good connection. Confusing because I never said no. Confusing because there were parts of it that were pleasurable. Confusing because I ultimately had an orgasm. Confusing because it wasn't something I wanted. Confusing because he was twenty years older and an authority figure to me.

Not much later, while I was living in Greenwich Village in New York City, a guy about my age started trying to court me. I remember him coming by the store where I worked, bringing me a fancy, overpriced cupcake, and wanting to take me out. I didn't know what to do with it. I still didn't feel anything that I considered attraction to other men but thought that maybe I should just go with it. At least this time, I could be *choosing* to explore a homoerotic experience, so, despite some hesitancy, I did. And all in all, it was a good experience. While it didn't blow my mind, it did feel like I was taking my power back. He was sweet, caring, and concerned about my consent and choice. I was trying to figure out my sexuality now that it had been put into question by the experience that had been thrust upon me.

When I walked into a room, I never felt a primary drive toward men like I did toward women, yet now I had a couple of experiences with other men under my belt, even if the first had left me head fucked. I spent years exploring the wide range of my sexual expression. In many ways, I still do. It is hard to look back at that first experience more than twenty years later and simply condemn it. In some ways it opened me up further.

Like most men, I grew up internalizing homophobia. Being perceived as gay was the worst thing in the world that could happen. It is tempting to look back at that first experience solely as one of violation, an experience that fucked me up and caused me to spend years trying to figure out my sexuality. Though that is all true, I can also look back at it as the catalyst that forced me to move through my internalized homophobia, the catalyst that opened me up to explore my sexuality beyond any preconceived confines. In this sense, the experience left an indelible and important mark on my path to becoming the Erotic Rockstar.

I think with most men, especially those born before 1980, the 100 percent heterosexual path is the easier path, yet I did a lot of exploring. I explored women. I explored men. I explored trans individuals. I have played with an intersexed individual. There is basically nobody of any type of sexual orientation or gender expression whom I didn't explore. I explored the full range of possibility, pushing more into the sense that my orientation was anything I hadn't already experienced. If I hadn't done it before, sure, let's try it. "Try-sexual" was my orientation of choice.

In many ways, that early experience helped invoke this dynamic erotic exploration. In other ways, it left me feeling fucked up. Still, twenty years later, it affects my relationship with Seth. It is tricky also because I like and care about him. Over these twenty years, he has shown up for me in many different ways. I have seen him grow on a personal level. I have seen him struggle with his homosexuality, and a decade later, I watched as he came out to his family and the world. I saw him marry his husband. I have witnessed his process and his growth.

One of the things that I find so challenging about the consent conversation as we are having it in larger society is that we like to make everything black and white. We like to villainize people and believe them to be monsters. We like to have bad guys we can drag through the mud. I don't think things are so clearly black and white. I have had twenty years to process this distinctly gray area with Seth, twenty years to get to know the man beyond one isolated experience. I now recognize that Seth was struggling with his own sexual identity.

At the time of my violation, President Bill Clinton had just signed the Defense of Marriage Act into law the year before, which defined marriage as being specifically between a man and a woman—an intentional slap in the face of queer Americans. In the midst of these political events, Seth was a man struggling to figure out how to be in a society and world that wasn't very friendly to people who had desires like he had. When desires are repressed, they come out in unhealthy ways. He had to move through his own internalized homophobia, and then I needed to move through mine.

Nonetheless, there was a clear power imbalance and clear intent on his part to get me drunk and stoned. Some would say he did so in order to have his way with me, and true, but also I believe it was to overcome his own shit. Again, I no longer hold any enmity toward him. Holding on to anger is hard when I can now experience compassion, empathy, and understanding. Still, it was wrong and had a very real impact on me.

I am not trying to encourage you to have sex with other men (nor discourage, you for that matter). Homophobia is about much more than another man's cock; much of it is about gendered expression. Are you fitting into and living up to a particular set of notions of what a man is "supposed to be"? I have come to recognize homophobia as having its roots in our fear of and devaluing of the feminine. Intense questioning of my sexuality led me to a point of IDGAF (I don't give a fuck) about other people's judgments of my sexuality. What I didn't expect was the incredible freedom that opened up in me. The more I was able to break free of any fears I had about other people's perceptions of my sexuality, the freer I felt to explore my broader humanity, including my inner feminine, and ultimately to figure out who I am and how I want to express myself in the world.

Despite how normative it is in American society today for men to restrict their choices and actions out of fear of being perceived as gay, is that really masculine? I don't believe masculinity is about making choices out of fear of other people's opinions. Masculinity has long been connected to a drive toward freedom. Living within a prison of homophobia is not freedom. You deserve to be free.

What stories do you have from your past that you don't want to tell? What has the impact been? In what ways do you carry homophobia? What would you do if you weren't afraid of being perceived as gay? What would change in your life if you were to fully break out of the prison of homophobia?

15.
GROUND AND CONNECT TO YOUR BODY

Despite my challenging family dynamic and difficulties with socializing with other kids in school, as a child I was consistently awarded positive feedback for my intellect. It was therefore natural for me to put more and more of my attention on my intelligence. In middle school, however, I started doing after-school sports, in part so I could spend longer periods of time away from the chaos of my home.

At fifteen, as the scrawny kid on the wrestling team, I had a debilitating injury. Picture eighty thirteen- to fifteen-year-old middle-school wrestlers in a gymnasium and the coach running over from the opposite side of the room because he heard something. That "something" was my back. We were running practice drills, and in that particular rotation, I was paired with one of our star wrestlers. As soon as the whistle blew, he pancaked me, grabbing me and slamming me down—which was normal and fine, except something had gone horribly wrong this time. In that testosterone-filled, traditional masculine environment, though I was guided to sit out for the remainder of that day, I was asked to come back in for the one-hundred-jumping-jack cool-down. Bouncing up and down on my feet, creating compression on my spine right after that injury, wasn't the smartest thing to do. I hobbled home that night in intense physical pain, not yet aware that the next decade of my life was going to be severely impacted by what had occurred in that dank middle-school gym.

I went to a doctor, who told me, "Sorry, kid, you are going to have your good days and your bad days. Your good days, well, good! Your bad days, well, you're just going to have to learn to get through them." At the age of fifteen, I learned and took on the belief that *I am now broken. There's nothing I can do. That's just how it is. My body is broken now. Deal with it.* I believed this prognosis for the next twelve years, experiencing both good days and bad days so painful that they would leave me bedridden—exactly as the doctor had predicted.

Over the next twelve years, my body continued to break down. I developed all sorts of compensatory patterns in the ways I moved my body as I learned to avoid pain. I didn't realize that was what I was doing, of course. What started in my mid-back spread to my low back, upper back, neck, hips, and knees. I reached a point of chronic pain at which there was never a moment that something wasn't hurting me. I couldn't remember anymore what it was like to not be in pain.

One of my first girlfriends in high school was all about us trading massages. I eventually realized that despite my body's deep need for relief, she was getting the better end of the deal. I learned over time that I had quite a knack for bodywork.

In 2003, trying to find a way to put myself through grad school, I attended a one-hundred-hour Swedish massage training. One of my classmates lived a short walking distance from my home in San Francisco, and we started meeting twice a week. Once a week, I would work on him for ninety minutes, and on another day he would work on me. In that process, I started to recognize the chronic tension I was holding in my body. I was completely unaware of how much my body was in a state of gripping, constant tension patterns. I even came to realize that much of my svelte body was created by my musculature intensely squeezing and spasming (which made sense given that I wasn't actually able to exercise with any regularity).

Something else unexpected also started to happen. I began to *feel* in my body—and in doing so, I was startled to realize how disconnected I was and that I hadn't been inhabiting my body for years. However, the thorn in that rose was that starting to feel sensation in my body also meant that I had to confront feeling the pain I had largely separated myself from. That was not fun, to say the least.

In 2005, I did my first ten-day Vipassana meditation sit. Imagine for a moment being woken up by a gong being struck at four in the morning, only to then sit on a cushion in seated meditation all day, until you go to sleep around eight-thirty at night. The next morning, the gong strikes at four o'clock, and the process starts all over again. Rinse and repeat for ten days. While it may sound like sitting all day is no big deal, let me tell you that sitting in stillness and silence for ten days is one of the most profoundly confronting experiences people can have in their lifetime.

I was prepared for a certain degree of psychological thrashing, but by far the most challenging thing about the experience was the excruciating shooting nerve pain that left me wild-eyed from one moment to the next. Prior to that, I was never sitting still. I was constantly in motion, fidgeting my body, because it was precisely how I kept myself from hurting so much.

The training was sequential, and by Day 4, the practice was one of not moving *at all*. In other words, if your leg falls asleep, you just surrender to being with it being asleep. If your nose itches, you are invited to observe the sensation of the itch arising, observe the itch for as long as it continues, and observe the itch sensation as it passes away. This totally kicked my ass—and was absolutely powerful for me.

I remember a particular point during a lunch break when there was a rare opportunity to break the silence and speak to one of the assistant teachers if we had an urgent need to do so. I approached the teacher with my question. "What do I do about this pain? This feels impossible for me."

The assistant teacher calmly said to me, "Sooner or later, you are going to have to learn how to be with the pain." My primal, instantaneous inner reaction was *Fuck you! You have no idea what I'm going through.* It took me years to understand what he was expressing to me and to see that he was right.

Two years later, I finally hit a breaking point and decided that I was not going to complain about my pain anymore. I was going to channel every ounce of energy I was putting into being upset about or complaining about my pain into actively healing my body. I had no idea that I had just arrived at a game-changing moment in my life.

I lived in the San Francisco Bay Area at the time, which had a flourishing healing arts community. I explored everything I could find, from focused massage and bodywork, acupuncture, and the Alexander Technique to the Feldenkrais Method and less widely known esoteric modalities. I began to develop a keen awareness of what I was doing with my body. I began to notice the tension patterns I was holding in my body and the inefficient, compensatory ways I had been moving it, from the most subtle to the most overt.

Step by step, I began to reprogram myself and how I used my body. Through focused attention, I became increasingly aware of unnecessary physical tension patterns and learned to let them go. For example, when I drove, all I needed to do was move my right foot between the gas and brake pedals. Simple enough—and yet my entire left leg was braced and my back muscles were squeezed tight, like they were holding on for dear life. I began to understand that there were many seemingly unrelated reasons why my body was hurting so much. I learned to find and feel into the tense parts of my body and to use deep breaths and long exhales to help me intentionally release the tension from where I was holding it.

The process of learning about the unconscious holding patterns in my own body was a powerful step in my realization of how much transformational change is possible—and hidden just out of view. Everything in my belief system prior to this point had taught me that if you have an injury like I did, you just learn to live with it for the rest of your life. I watch my brother-in-law do just that: ten years ago, he had a back injury while working his warehouse job, and ever since, he has just learned to live with it. Over the years, I have watched him stuff himself down to a smaller expression of himself in order to stoically press on and live with the pain. For nearly half my life, I had been doing the same thing.

Whether through incessant physical pain or simply the ways in which the intellect is praised over the body, many men learn—just as I had—to dissociate from the body. Escaping the body like this may help with ignoring the pain, but it is at the price of decreasing our ability to experience pleasure. In other words, when we dissociate from the body because the pain is so great, we also lose touch with our emotions, the communications of the body, and our capacity to feel pleasure.

As I began to anchor into my body again, I found it easier to stop experiencing the world solely through intellectually analyzing and mentally understanding it. I began experiencing the world by being present in my animal body and my five senses. The more I became present in my body, the more I felt like I was interfacing with reality instead of my *ideas* about reality.

Much of what I learned through my lived experience during this process mapped onto my approach of sexual self-mastery. As I learned to attune to my body and observe what was going on within it, I began to notice subtleties that I had been completely unaware of. I was able to extend this awareness of the subtlety of sensation within my own body into a deepening awareness of subtleties that were going on in other people's bodies. This informed and laid the foundation for the sexual attunement processes I used to create powerful experiences with women (as described in Part IV: "Understanding Women and the Feminine").

This transformation of my body also showed me that there is far more possible with respect to creating radical change in one's life than I had believed. Through this recognition, I started bringing that belief to more areas of my life.

Initially, I held the belief that I just had to deal with having a broken body. *This is just how I am due to what happened in the past.* My identity was in my wound and in what the world inflicted on me. After an intense journey spurred on by this crisis, I arrived at a point that would eventually lead me to create a new set of beliefs based on the reality of my own experience: *I can create my life, even my body. I can transform it. I can create my future. And it starts right now.*

> How grounded and connected do you feel to your body? Have you learned to numb yourself to your body in pursuit of your career or an "ideal" body, or because of pain or some other reason? What will change in your life as you become a deeply grounded and connected man?

16.
CULTIVATE DEEP PRESENCE

Presence is the difference between an invisible man leading a life of "quiet desperation" (as Thoreau wrote in *Walden*) and a man who turns heads as he walks into a room. I have come to think of presence as the cornerstone of masculine potency and power. When someone says or thinks, "There's something different about this man," whether they are aware of it or not, they are likely picking up on his capacity to be *present*.

Being present means not being in your mind chatter, not being in anxiety, fear, or fantasy. Presence means not worrying about the past or what has happened before, or being concerned about what might happen. Presence is not worrying about how she is going to react or if you are doing this right. It is not trying to plan the next move or wondering what you are supposed to say. All of those things have you up in your head. Being present is being in your body and connected to your five senses: sight, hearing, touch, taste, and smell.

When you are in your five senses, you are not in your mind. You are present in the moment. Women are incredibly sensitive to this presence, even though many wouldn't necessarily be able to articulate it. They can sense when you are present with them, and likewise, they can sense when you are not. They can sense when you are up in your head, when you are anxious or fearful, and when you are somewhere else. Quite simply, these are turnoffs.

Men have come to me many times and said things like, "I don't understand what her problem is. Yeah, I was getting something done on my computer, but I was still listening." No. That's never going to work. What she is aching for is to feel you in that moment, and she feels you in that moment when you have the fullness of your presence, the fullness of your attention, *on her*.

One key to presence is attention, the second is being connected to your five senses. The third is being in your body.

The first story I am going to share with you is not my own. It is a composite of stories told to me over and over again by women I have loved as friends and as lovers.

> I was having sex with my boyfriend. One moment we felt incredibly connected, and I was on the edge of what felt like was going to be a powerful orgasm, and the next moment, I could suddenly feel that even though he was still physically inside of me, he was gone. I could feel and hear his mind chatter—it went from making love to a mechanical act. Suddenly feeling abandoned and betrayed, I became sad and angry, closed my legs, and told him to get off of me. I started to cry.

> To be so close to and opened by a man—creating a deep sexual experience together—*and then having him gone,* just checked out, made me feel crazy. Even though we talked about it many times, it took me a long time to feel safe enough to open to him that deeply again. I wish men knew how important being present is for a woman—and how hurtful it is when they aren't present, especially when having sex.

Women and sex were both my inspiration and my training ground to cultivate my ability to stay fully present. Women are primal huntresses for masculine presence. They will track you and your capacity to be and stay present the way a lion stalks a gazelle in the early morning light. If you want to open a woman into the fullness of her desire—wet, hot, and hungry for you—you need to build your capacity for presence.

Presence can appear and be revealed in life in many different ways. In 2002, at twenty-four years old, I attended Burning Man for the first time. There, hung along the walls of Center Camp, was a sign that read: "You are not your thoughts, you are that which observes your thoughts." *What does that even mean,* I wondered. I had spent my entire life being praised for my thoughts and my ability to think them. I had also experienced times of feeling like the incessant chatter of my mind was driving me insane. As a young man with a mental velocity that unintentionally blew others (and my own self) out of the water, the sign's message invoked a feeling I can only describe as a cosmic mind fuck.

Flash forward three years: The cool air coming into my nostrils and warm air coming out across my upper lip was where I was placing the entirety of my attention. This was very difficult for me to focus on at the time because the relentless mental chatter was far more pronounced than any sensation on my lip. Sometime on Day 5 of that first ten-day Vipassana meditation retreat, I had a hallelujah moment. Suddenly, n-o-t-h-i-n-g—an experience that I can only describe as peace. Since I had always been ADHD-oriented and probably on the bipolar spectrum with radically turbulent energy and emotion, that moment of peace felt like nirvana—and I just wanted more.

Luckily, I had five days left, and the experience of peace went much deeper still. I left there with a new direction to point myself in. It was a peak experience, like doing MDMA for the first time, where you have this heightened experience that gives you a glimpse of possibility, and then you drop back into "not that," but your world is forever changed. Now I had real lived experience of complete stillness of my mind and true presence of being. I had heard such things spoken of, but I certainly hadn't been able to understand them. It hadn't been real to me by any means. But now it was *real*—and I wanted more, so I started bringing more attention into actively cultivating it. My world was forever changed.

(Pro tip: If I had known how deeply meditation would change my sex life for the better, I would have started years earlier.)

From the walls of Center Camp at Burning Man to two ten-day Vipassana meditation retreats, to launching a seven-year epic hero's journey as the Erotic Rockstar, to building The Evolved Masculine—a thriving company coaching hundreds of men annually—I am more clear than ever that presence is *the* underlying cornerstone to creating multifaceted success in a man's life.

> How present are you, really? As you quiet down your mental chatter and learn to find stillness and be present in your body, what impact do you believe this will have on the man you are becoming?

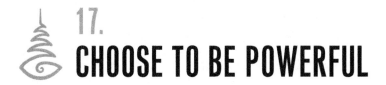

17.
CHOOSE TO BE POWERFUL

I believe that the entire energetic signature of "masculine power" is in a state of deep evolutionary reorganization in our culture. The writing is on the wall: the form of power that has been a fuel source for men in the Western world is in the midst of a massive collective shakedown. The type of power that men have used to get them "here" simply will not get them "there." In many ways, this reorganization of male power has been catalyzed by the rising of the Feminine. As women and that which we know as "the Feminine" (as explored in Part IV, "Understanding Women and the Feminine") reclaim their inherent potency, it is demanded that masculine power evolve and mature at a velocity not seen in our lifetime.

Nearly all men can stand adversity, but if you
want to test a man's character, give him power.

— Abraham Lincoln

For many years, I held a negative association with the word *power*. Our history and current reality is teeming with examples of the ways in which power has been abused in the hands of the men who wield it. Power meant taking what you want regardless of who got hurt in the process. From that negative association, it was clear to me that I didn't want to be *that*, so I dimmed my own power—and my *desire* for power—out of fear of being or becoming the very thing I despised.

Now, in the wake of the #metoo movement, more and more men have been doing the same. Afraid of their own power, many men, especially younger men, are cutting off connection from a vital part of their masculine essence. This is a form of energetic self-castration, and despite its understandable arrival, it is actually a *symptom* of the wound, not a solution.

Historically, we have been focused on an old hierarchical dominance paradigm of *power over*: my power in relation to yours; my ability to dominate and bend you to my will. The Evolved Masculine has eschewed this distorted power-over approach of the past. He has seen the damage this way of being has inflicted on women, children, the planet, and even on ourselves as men. True power is sourced from within. It is not something that can be given, nor can it be taken away. In this sense, personal empowerment is your core essence coming into its fullest expression. Since coming to this definition, I have aimed to ever and ongoingly increase my power.

This has nothing to do with anyone else. It is your journey and your journey alone. This type of power is one in which the more empowered you are, the more others naturally feel more empowered in your presence.

As we let our own light shine, we unconsciously give other people permission to do the same.

— Marianne Williamson

It may seem strange to focus on empowering men when there are so many examples of men abusing their power, but I have come to believe that these abuses are rooted in an internal feeling of powerlessness, and from that place of powerlessness comes an overcompensation and a compulsive need to constantly prove one's power.

Far too much harm has been done by men who were trying to prove to the world, to other men, and to themselves that they were "real men." When we are connected to our true power, there is nothing to prove. It is certainly not about making others feel less than. On the contrary, others feel like they rise up in the presence of men in their true power; they are more of who they are capable of being. They feel like they have more choice available to them. They are capable of doing more in the world. They feel more empowered and free around these men.

I realized that if I am not happy with the way in which others wield their power, then I could either spend my life living at the effect of what other "more powerful" people do and simply complain about it, or I could actively and intentionally cultivate my own power and help show a better way. Choosing to be powerful requires that I trust myself with the responsibility that comes with that power.

To be powerful requires you to stand in your power, your value, your worth, and your capacity. By doing so, you are intrinsically inspiring and inviting others to rise up in their own power, as well.

I can recall a specific moment more than a decade ago in which I wrote these words on a piece of paper to pin to my vision cork board:

— *Choose to be Powerful!* —

I remember the energy that coursed through me as I wrote it. *Can I do that? Is that OK? Is that possible?* In that moment, I did. I made a choice. I chose to be powerful. Over the years, that choosing came to fruition. As I cultivated my truth, my voice, my power, and my potency more and more, day by day, year by year, I became an empowered, powerful man, and it all started with a decision.

One of the most essential core principles of the Evolved Masculine path is that men must form a healthy relationship to their power. Collapsing or avoiding the responsibility of your power is part of the problem. Continuing the distorted and dying dominance paradigm while hiding behind a nice-guy smile is equally as problematic to not just your self but also to women and the world. In order to be on the path of the Evolved Masculine, you must cultivate a conscious understanding of the rightness of your power as a man. Despite the prominence of messaging saying otherwise, I believe that our broken world does not need less masculine power, we need *more* men in right relationship to their masculine power.

> What is your relationship to power? Do you chase it? Do you fear it? Do you trust yourself to use power wisely? What would a healthy relationship to power be like for you? Are you ready to choose to be powerful?

18.
BE A MAN OF INTEGRITY

When I first found the tantra and sacred sexuality community, I thought I had finally found the solution I had been looking for. Here was a whole community of people who were talking about, and seemingly addressing, sexual trauma. My background in massage and training as a certified sexological bodyworker laid a strong foundation for the types of hands-on sexual healing that the community was built on.

Shortly after my completion of the sexological bodyworker training and certification in 2006, I went to a daka-dakini tantra conference in Sedona, Arizona. (*Daka* and *dakini* are the male and female forms of the word used for a tantric sexual healer and practitioner.) I quickly noticed how wildly different the two lineages were in terms of how they addressed the complex subject of sexual trauma. Whereas the sexological bodyworker profession placed a high importance on creating a professional distance between practitioner and client, tantric practice did not. The sexological bodyworkers had strict codes of ethics that included the practitioner always staying fully clothed, wearing gloves for all genital and anal touch, and placing the emphasis on the client and their connection to their own body and sexuality and away from any connection with the practitioner.

The approach among tantric practitioners was quite the opposite. Dakas and dakinis intentionally utilized creating a feeling of deep connection and intimacy between practitioner and client, holding the belief that the experience of profound intimacy is itself a healing act. The emphasis on intimacy and connection held heightened value in the eyes of the tantric practitioners because many people don't have a map in their system of that level of connection and intimacy. The tantric community believed that by having a lived experience of deep human connection within a safe container, the client would leave with an imprint with which to be able to recreate deeper intimacy in their relationships moving forward.

Given my history with intimacy being the one place where I found solace in a world that I felt never understood me, the ability to create intimate connection was a superpower of mine. The idea of using this capacity that I held in service to others really drew me. (Admittedly, the fact that this community felt sexy and fun, with hot tub gatherings, casual nudity, and dance parties, only added to its magnetism.)

It wasn't just all hot tub parties and sensual dance, however. During the first daka-dakini conference I attended, its founder, Forest Roberts, was being accused of sexually assaulting one of his clients. I didn't know people in this community yet, but the alleged assault was already touching my hot-button issue. Although the matter was never settled, I always looked at this person askance and held him at a certain distance. Right out of the gate, it demonstrated to me the tragic irony inherent in a lineage devoted to sacred sexuality: that it may contain the very thing it is also attempting to heal. Nonetheless, despite these serious misgivings, over time I increased my involvement in the organization that Forest helped build.

Over the course of the next few years, I rose in prominence in this global community and brought what I learned through sexological bodywork and other trainings into the teachings I shared. My Erotic Rockstar persona, with my eccentric attire and strong personality, turned heads, while my commitment to bold leadership and finding deeper truths delivered value.

Over time, it became clear that I was seeing what struck me as a lack of integrity in the community, particularly among much of the leadership. The dark side of sexual healing was being illuminated, and ironically, many in leadership were more focused on their own sexual gratification than on the stated aims of global sexual healing.

Looking back, I believe that the ethical foundations that were built into the sexological bodywork training, along with the profound impact of Anjali's rape, helped inoculate me against the predatory behaviors I often saw in the tantra community. It was amazing to me that while there was always talk about this leader's "shadow," nothing was ever done about it. I was really impacted by people's refusal to look at these serious concerns or to even engage in the conversations when they were brought up. This avoidance and denial of the palpable knowledge that there was something rotten in the organization always felt like an even larger and more problematic integrity issue.

It became clear that the sacred sexuality community had a bad reputation among the larger spiritual/conscious community world. I came to believe that much of their dicey reputation was well deserved. It would not be enough for the tantra community to clean up its messes and stop its integrity violation issues—which they were not even doing at the time. The only solution that I could see would be for the sacred sexuality community to become *models of sexual integrity*. To gain any standing in the world and hope to have the impact the leaders claim to care about, they would have to become the beacon that other communities could look to in order to learn how to do things right and be with one's sexuality with integrity.

Ultimately, I learned much about integrity, and the lack thereof, through the sacred sexuality community. I had the unfortunate opportunity to intimately witness the wide array of problems that arise when one doesn't prioritize integrity.

These complex experiences helped me to see the importance of walking your talk, getting clear on what your values and principles are, and living in alignment with them—even when it doesn't feel good or requires you to go beyond what is comfortable. It is not enough to simply speak or teach about what you believe in; rather, true leadership requires you to be a *living example* of what you believe in.

My time in the sacred sexuality community came to a head when the Global Tantra Alliance (GTA) was courting me to potentially take over, as Forest Roberts was going into semi-retirement; GTA even organized an Australia-Bali teaching tour for me. In the midst of a week-long sacred sexuality intensive, I met an amazing woman, Allison, whom I can best describe as not just being a radiant spirit but also the most versatile lover I had ever had. I quickly found out that she had just ended a lovership with Forest.

Allison and I started our romantic connection while she was still processing her relationship with Forest. I would hear how she spoke to her friends in detail about her experience with him and the impact that his half-truths and rampant promiscuity had on her. I could feel the pain and impact his behavior had on her. I cringed at the idea of a woman speaking about my behavior negatively impacting her like that. I saw the ways in which living my life the way I was living it, I was going to be just like Forest in twenty years. *I could see the ways in which I already was.*

One day, after a full day of leading sex workshops, Forest came back to the place we were both staying at with a local event organizer, and there was a moment in which I saw what I swear I could describe only as loneliness in his eyes. I saw that though he had a certain kind of male fantasy life—traveling around the world, teaching about sex and intimacy, having a woman in every port—and that most of these women were a good twenty years younger than him, everything was so transient. At the end of the day, he didn't have that lifelong companion to share his world with. Whether I read too much into that moment or not, it hit me deep. *I don't think this is what I want.*

I knew in that moment that I couldn't further consider taking over leadership of the organization. I was all set up to follow in his footsteps, and in fact, I was already living much of the same lifestyle, yet when I saw the path before me through his reflection, it was obvious that I had gone down that road as far as I was going to go. But, damn, being immersed in the community, I was surrounded by beautiful, sexually open women; I received constant attention and adulation while I traveled around the world having erotic adventures. Was I really going to give all *that* up?!

Despite all the sexy glamour of what that opportunity had to offer me, it wasn't in alignment with my Evolved Masculine self, who was already beginning to emerge. I decided to let it go in order to gain clarity on what would be congruent with my principles and values. That moment of surrendering my egoic desire in order to align with my deeper knowing was an apex of choosing my own integrity even when the cost *appeared* to be high.

As seductive as the opportunity appeared on the surface, however, there wasn't really anything to be lost. In fact, I was being set up to gain something much greater. I have come to believe that when we align with our integrity, there is only something to gain, despite how the circumstances may appear on the surface. Integrity is a foundational principle of the Evolved Masculine path. The Evolved Masculine must be willing to move beyond what is comfortable for him in order to do that which he believes is right. It does not matter what the cost is, there is nothing more important to the soul of a man than his own personal integrity.

What are your principles and values? In what ways are you living in accordance to them? In what ways are you not? What would you be willing to give up in order to hold on to your integrity?

19.
PROTECT THE FEMININE

It was New Year's Eve, 2007. Kirsten and I were performing at Sea of Dreams, a ten-thousand-person event in San Francisco. It was by far the biggest public performance I had done with her. She did a trapeze act twenty-five feet up in the air. In the upstairs VIP area, she and I did a combination lap dance/pole dance/acro balance duet together that we had been working on for months. We followed it with a sword-and-contact-juggling duo performance inside of a giant inflatable snow globe about a story high, way above the crowd of many thousands of people, during Thievery Corporation's set. It was, in a word, *phenomenal.*

At the end of the long night, we met an extremely charismatic man named Yuri, who had a very strong and intense energy. He invited us back to his place, tempting us by saying that he had an infinity pool set to 104 degrees—perfect hot tub temperature.

Wow.

Given that Kirsten and I were both novelty junkies, constantly seeking new adventures, it was a no brainer that we would go. On the drive to his place (with one of his minions driving), he was sitting in the back with us, scraping sassafras (organic Ecstasy) off of a crystalline rock with a knife and giving it to us in hefty doses.

This was yet another new experience I eagerly—and literally—gobbled up. By the time we arrived to his place, we were both already "rolling" hard—rave lingo for being deep inside the Ecstasy. We arrived at his place and immediately understood that this man was a total baller. There were half a dozen people wandering around the house who appeared to be his crew, and it was clear that he was the head honcho. His place was opulent. The crappy little one-bedroom apartment that Kirsten and I shared could have easily fit in his living room—with room to spare.

We sat down just as Yuri began rolling a joint. We were high to the point of becoming disoriented but feeling oh-so-good. The next thing I am able to recall is Yuri climbing all over us, making out with both of us. I would look over to check on Kirsten; she seemed to be having a great time, so I continued to go along with it. Slowly, Yuri became more aggressive and was clearly trying to push things toward sex.

I could sense that Kirsten was a hard no, which honestly relieved me, but Yuri didn't pick up on it—either he didn't notice or didn't care. Instead, he was so intent on getting what he wanted that he was unconcerned about our needs and desires.

It reached a breaking point when I literally had to push him away and off of Kirsten. He stopped for a few moments and then started trying to climb on top of us while nately attempting to yank down her or my pants. I could feel Kirsten starting to shut down. As he became more aggressive toward us, I became more aggressive in my pushback. He would back off and engage in casual conversation with us only to leap back onto us once more, clawing at our clothes. He seemed to believe that all he had to do was stop for a minute or two and then just go right back after what he wanted, regardless of the consistent display of our boundaries. This is my most direct experience with being on the receiving end of a man's persistence in the face of a clear no, in line with the intensely troubling stories I have heard from so many women.

This is a prime example of the problem that can arise when men are taught that we are supposed to be the constant driving force toward sex. The narrative that has been taught and rewarded in our society is that it is "our job to make it happen" and that any resistance from her is just a token expression that she musters up so you don't think she is a slut. Some men are taught that this "token resistance" is like a challenge, that it is simply something we are supposed to get around so that we can get what we want without thinking less of her and her sexual appetite.

I felt Kirsten shut down. If I hadn't been there, I can only imagine that she would have frozen (as she was already starting to do)—which is a common automatic defense mechanism triggered in the face of a threatening situation—and that he would have raped her. And chances are, in his mind, he wouldn't have thought he had done anything wrong.

Unfortunately, the story doesn't end there. Having spent so much of my life being raised in a blue-collar working-class family that always struggled to get by, and then once off on my own having lived around the poverty line for another decade after that, I was enamored by Yuri's wealth. I was both fascinated by and fearful of the power he held. It was like being starstruck—I was in constant observation of and seduced by the way the people around him looked to him, followed him, and did what he said.

Despite that extremely questionable experience, we continued to get together with Yuri over the next couple of months. There were always lots of high-quality drugs flowing, all provided by him. He took care of and paid for everything. He didn't try to engage with us physically again; it was more like we were folded into being part of his posse as his own personal entertainment.

One time, when we were all together hanging out in Yuri's grandiose home, we brought my dear friend Jacklyn with us. Once again, Yuri was doling out massive doses of his famous sassafras, possibly even larger amounts this time. The drugs were so strong that we could barely move, and our eyes were vibrating and rolling back into our heads. We were rolling extremely intensely, riding wave after wave of wild ecstasy and euphoria while being in a complete stupor. At one point, Yuri grabbed Jacklyn's hand and began to lead her away. I remember feeling discomfort in that moment but thinking to myself, *Jacklyn's her own person. She makes her own choices. It is not my right to interfere, and this has nothing to do with me.* I kept my focus on Kirsten, making sure she was okay.

Even though I told myself it was not my place to intervene, the fact was that *it was my responsibility.* Jacklyn was at his home for one reason only: I had invited her, and she trusted me. Of course, that night he did the same thing with her that he did when I first met him: he filled her with drugs to the point of total incapacitation and then tried to fuck her.

It is now ten years later, and Jacklyn still doesn't know what happened that night. She doesn't have any memories beyond flashes of him trying to touch her pussy while she feebly tried to push his hand away, but being so fucked up, she couldn't really move. Other than that, her memories are blank. She says that not knowing if she was raped that night fucks with her head even more than the time when she knows clearly that she was raped.

I failed Jacklyn that night. My education and beliefs at the time around equality and sameness between men and women had me denying any sense of role or responsibility as a man. As a result, a woman I deeply cared about may have been raped on my watch. I swore to myself: never again. Even today, I can feel the emotional anguish of having failed to show up and own that critical evolutionary male role of the protector.

Never again.

Some time later, I went to a house party of about a hundred and fifty people in the Mission District of San Francisco. I ran into Jacklyn there, and she excitedly told me that she wanted to introduce me to a guy named Daniel whom she was starting to get to know. Daniel came by a few minutes later, and my alarm bells immediately went off. I had seen Jacklyn with various men over the course of our multi-year friendship, and I had never experienced anything like this. Something inside of me was screaming *Danger!* After a brief hello, he quickly went on his way.

I sat with that discomfort in my body. I didn't see him for the rest of the party until the end of the night. Jacklyn and I had decided to share a cab back to the other side of the city together, as we lived walking distance apart. As we were heading down to the street from the party, I found out that Daniel was joining us in the cab ride to go back to Jacklyn's place. I did not like this.

We were sitting in the taxi cab, with Jacklyn in the middle and Daniel and me flanking her on either side. I was checking in with myself: *Is this jealousy? I don't think so. This is very different from anything I've felt about any other man she's been with.*

I said to her as discreetly as I was able, "You know, you don't have to do this. You don't have to take him home with you."

She responded, "Oh, I don't know. Daniel doesn't listen to me."

I shot back, "That does not make me feel any better."

Despite my attempt at discretion, Daniel clearly overheard me and started to become irate. "Who the fuck do you think you are?" he yelled at me. "Where I'm from, interfering like that is asking for a fight. You wanna fight?"

"No man, I don't want to fight, but I'm not comfortable with you going home with her, either," I responded as calmly as I could.

He then reached over Jacklyn to try to take a swing at me. I parried as he tried a few more times. "Stop it, man. You're going to hurt her!" I exclaimed.

"I don't fucking care!" he yelled back.

I glared at him, "Exactly, man. *Exactly*."

I heard the taxi driver calling the police as Daniel's physical aggression continued to escalate. I could tell that everything in his body wanted to fight. As I tried to de-escalate the situation and physically block Jacklyn from inadvertently getting hurt, we could hear the approaching police sirens. Just as we saw the flashing lights coming toward us, Daniel jumped out of the taxi and disappeared into the night.

We had the taxi take us both back to my place. When we got up to the apartment, Jacklyn started to unleash on me. "How dare you? Who do you think you are? You had no right. I'm fucking pissed off at you." I felt bewildered, as it was so obvious and clear to me that I did what needed to be done.

I told her, "Look, Jacklyn, I don't care if you hate me and don't ever want to see me again. I'm still really glad that I did what I did and intervened." Though she reacted very strongly in the moment, in the weeks afterward, she expressed gratitude and what felt like a heightened respect for me.

There is a reason why men throughout history have taken on the role of protector: there are rapists and violent men in our midst who have no intention of changing. I recognize that this piece is a knife's edge because the very reason we need more men to be inspired protectors of women and the feminine is because there are *men* with very damaged relationships to their masculine who walk among us.

Yes, women are rising in their power. Yes, women have incredible strength of will and far greater capacity than we as a society have historically given them credit for, yet the masculine role of protector is not a role to give up. It has been distorted by many men who confuse protection with control and ownership.

However, there is a way that you can claim the role of protector in a manner that has her feel *more* free instead of less as a result.

Being a husband and father, I now take my role of protector very seriously. It is a responsibility that I willfully and joyfully take on. I choose to hold the responsibility to keep my family safe, to keep an eye on the environment that we are in, in a state of relaxed vigilance. I am highly aware, but I am not tense.

In owning my role of protector, I feel a responsibility to know how to protect and defend my family, those I care about, and those in my charge. The moment it crosses over into control is the moment that the Evolved Masculine protector has ceased and the toxic masculine power drive has come out.

I believe that providing protection for all beings who are more vulnerable than men—women, children, the elderly, and our planet—is an essential dimension of the Evolved Masculine. I believe that one of the greatest roles men can take on today is an evolved version of this protector role. The Evolved Masculine protector focuses on widening the container for her so she can feel safe to explore, to express, and to be. She should always feel more free in your presence as her protector, not less. It is the job of the Evolved Masculine to create a world in which all women feel safe: safe to feel free, to blossom, and to flourish.

What is your relationship to the role of protector? How have you neglected this role? How have you shown up in your past as the distorted protector? What course correction could you implement to step more potently into your own Evolved Masculine protector?

20.
CHOOSE TO FORGIVE YOUR FATHER

My relationship with my dad was very difficult when I was growing up. My dad worked as a mailman for the post office for thirty-five years. What was clear to me throughout my childhood was that he hated his job. He woke up at four o'clock every morning to commute for an hour in traffic. He worked all of the overtime he could, often putting in sixty-hour work weeks, to make sure that he could provide for his family.

What I knew was that he was almost never home, and when he was, he was miserable to be around: screaming at my mom, yelling at or hitting me, or sending me to my room, crying. For many years I just thought he was an asshole. When I was fifteen years old, my parents finally sat me and my sister down to tell us that they were separating. I just exclaimed out loud, "What took so fucking long?!"

Honestly, it was a huge relief for me when my dad left. For the next three years, by my own choice, I barely saw him. I harbored a lot of anger and resentment toward him and spent as little time with him as I could. Over the next few years, however, I couldn't help but notice that he wasn't the same man anymore. Separated from my equally unhappy mother and no longer living in the house where there was so much conditioned animosity, he began to change and soften.

Even after I became aware of this, it still took me another ten years to arrive at a place where I decided that I wanted to have a better relationship with my father. In that choice lay the difficult truth that if that was going to happen, it was going to be because *I* did something about it. In other words, if I wanted a better relationship with my father—the man who I had been so afraid of and had held such deep anger toward—it was going to be up to *me*.

I put in the work. I picked up the phone. I had what were initially extremely uncomfortable and awkward conversations—long silences and moments of searching for *something* we shared as a common interest to discuss. At first, there were many moments of struggling to find a way to create a connection beyond the superficial, but step by step, it got easier. It took me until my thirties to start expanding my understanding of the life of the man who was my father.

He had spent my childhood feeling trapped. He was in a loveless, sexless marriage with a woman he wasn't attracted to and usually didn't even get along with. He did everything he thought was expected of him or that he knew how to do. Despite his resentment, he went to work every damn day. He was our family's sole provider, and he poured every cent into us. He didn't spend any of the money he worked so hard for on himself, while making sure that my sister and I had all of the toys and childhood experiences we could ever want. This included providing for his wife, whom he didn't even really like.

Despite all this, through his lens, she wasn't keeping up her end of the unspoken bargain. She didn't work. She watched eight-plus hours of television a day while the house was in shambles, and she gained more and more weight. (While I can understand my father's increasing frustration and hostility, learning more about the effects of trauma has allowed me to access greater compassion for my mom, as will be addressed in chapter 43, "The First Woman You Will Ever Love.")

My father had lacked strong, positive male role models in his childhood, as well. His father was a raging alcoholic who died when my dad was twelve years old, leaving my dad as the man of the house to take care of his wheelchair-bound mother. While only a child, he was forced to learn to step into a place of responsibility, providing for and figuring out how to make the household work and make ends meet.

Though an intelligent man, my dad had to drop out of community college because he needed to work full time to take care of his mother. The job he got in his early twenties at the local post office to better support his disabled mother, which provided stability and security, was the same job he held for more than thirty-five years. My dad was never given the opportunity to live into his potential—nor did he have the resources to even imagine he could create something different, something better.

It is now, with compassion, that I can imagine he felt like life was one compromise after another. This is the invisible role that consumes so many men: the stoic soldiering on, waking up every day at an ungodly hour, spending the next twelve hours commuting or working at an unfulfilling job with supervisors who demean you.

Because of his sacrifice, I can literally only imagine the feeling of such intense powerlessness, both at work and in the home life. It is a pressure cooker with no escape, either at work or home. I do not excuse, but I can understand the drivers that caused my father to exert and express what little power he had through his anger and rage at his family, trying to feel some semblance of control over his life. He sacrificed his own hopes and dreams to do that which was expected of him, year after year, despite not ever receiving any real satisfaction or fulfillment in return. What must this do to a man's spirit?

I do not condone all of the things my father did. I do not condone the way he yelled, screamed, and hit me throughout my childhood, such that I spent my childhood fearing him. I do not condone his punching that hole in the wall. I do not condone that time when, in the heat of an argument, he hit my mom, giving her a black eye. I will never condone those things. But at this point in my life, I have a better understanding of where they came from and how he came to be the way he was.

I see the changes in the man and how he shows up today. His diagnosis of prostate cancer changed and softened him. As he had to face his mortality, he came out the other side with a sense of gratitude for being here. Becoming a grandfather has changed him, first with my sister's two children, then with my own child. I love seeing him show up in the way that he wishes he had had the capacity to do when we were children. Being in retirement, no longer working, and living with my sister, he is able to be a daily part of his grandkids' lives, making up for missing our whole childhoods due to working all the time. Regardless of his changes, my forgiveness of him started first. At the end of the day, my forgiveness is less for him as it is for me.

As I learned to forgive my father, something in me relaxed and let go. I no longer hold anger or resentments toward my father at all, and with that comes a greater sense of peace as well as freedom.

I have taken on the belief that we are all doing the best we can with the resources that are available to us, and I have so much available to me that my father didn't have. I have so much available to me *because* of choices and sacrifices that my father made. I have also lived long enough to make plenty of mistakes of my own, to get in touch with my own shadow and dark side, and to learn how to forgive myself enough that I could forgive him. From that forgiveness, a new chapter of our relationship with one another could begin.

I have been around enough to know that life isn't promised. Tomorrow isn't promised. Hell, the rest of today isn't promised to anyone. I could either forgive and make peace with my father now, while he is alive, or be left trying to figure out how to find that peace after his death.

What stories do you hold around your father? Are you trying to prove yourself to him? Is some part of you still rebelling against him? What anger or resentments do you hold against your father? Who would you be if you were to choose forgiveness?

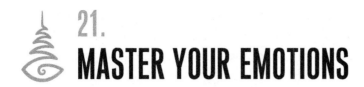

21.
MASTER YOUR EMOTIONS

After actively exploring my emotions for more than a decade, I still am able to cry only if I am in the arms of a woman I trust. There is something safe and nurturing about being held by a woman that gives me permission to let the tears flow. There are other times when I feel great grief in my body, and intellectually I know that crying would be really good for me and provide a release that my system needs. However, without that feminine presence, I am not able to cry beyond a slight moisture developing at the corners of my eyes. This is not innate, so why am I like this?

I did not have a good role model of what an emotionally healthy and expressed man was like. Many of us learn as boys that our emotions are not welcome. "Stop crying." "Don't be a sissy." "Man up." "Toughen up." "What are you, a faggot?" So I, like many boys growing up, learned to stuff those emotions. Not only don't cry, but don't smile too much, either. Don't trust your emotions. In fact, it's better not to feel them at all, so I learned to be stoic. As I started to rebel against my masculinity, however, I knew I didn't want to be shut down anymore, so I let myself feel, but too often, I also let my emotions rule me.

I spent many years reacting immediately to whatever emotion got stirred up in me. I didn't understand why I would hear so many women say they wished men would show their emotions more, even as my emotional expression was never welcomed or appreciated.

I have come to understand that while it doesn't help to suppress emotions, I can still learn healthier ways to *be* with them. The Latin root of emotion is *emotere*, which translates to "energy in motion." Learning to master my emotions was simply another aspect of mastering my energy.

The Evolved Masculine feels—and feels deeply—yet he is not controlled by his emotions, nor does he numb himself to them.

Yes, the emotions can be considered an aspect of the feminine part of our being. Integrate that shit. Making peace with your feminine, learning to appreciate it, and finding its strengths can make you a stronger man. Emotional mastery is about learning to simply *be* with the energy—neither shutting it down nor letting it run the show. Every emotion you feel has physical sensations that go along with it.

I remember when I was first exploring open relationships, my girlfriend was living in a different state, and though I had another regular lover, when my girlfriend started having sex with another man in her town, I freaked out. On an intellectual level, I understood that it was only fair, as I had already had other lovers (repeatedly) since we had gotten together. Emotionally, though, I didn't know how to handle it. I felt incredible jealousy.

Then I got curious about what feeling jealous actually meant. I began to notice the sensations in my body. I came to notice that when I felt jealous, I felt a heavy pressure in my chest, a tightening in my throat, and heat rising up through my head. Once I could identify what was happening physically, like I initially learned in Vipassana, I taught myself to simply observe the sensations without judgment.

I would watch these intense sensations knowing that as uncomfortable as they were, they weren't going to kill me. I observed all of the uncomfortable feelings in my body until they eventually went away on their own. The more I relaxed and just let myself be with the feelings, the more they started to feel more manageable. Noticing the emotions and learning to be with them allowed me to take clearer conscious action instead of simply being in unconscious reaction.

The methods I explored through my process of sexual self-mastery helped me to expand my capacity to both notice the subtle sensations that were happening in my body and to run more energy through my system without letting it release uncontrollably. I learned to hold the energy and let it move through me while grounding myself.

The Evolved Masculine is a master of his own emotions. This doesn't mean that he represses them. No, he knows how to feel, and feel fully, as he knows how to witness and be with his emotions. He can let the emotions move through his body and is able to choose how he responds. No longer a slave to his emotions, he doesn't react; rather, he has learned to listen to his emotions as teachers and guides. Each one has a message to share with him in the moment to better understand himself and his environment.

How connected are you to your emotions? What are you feeling right now? Do you need to learn to let yourself feel more? Or how to contain and be with your emotions more? Or both? How would emotional mastery improve the quality of your life?

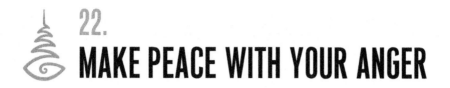

22.
MAKE PEACE WITH YOUR ANGER

I had a very hard time with my anger. I had a very hard time *having* anger. I hated my anger. I thought of my anger as my big flaw—evidence that there was something wrong with me. Beneath that was the deeper fear that perhaps I wasn't a good man after all.

I grew up in a household with a lot of anger, where rage flew often between my parents. It was a home where fighting with your loved one meant yelling, screaming, maybe even punching a hole in the wall. It was commonplace that emotions were expressed by doors slamming or cars screeching out the driveway.

These dysfunctional familial patterns followed me as I began to experience intense emotions, relationships, and falling in love. As much as I loved each woman I fell in love with and felt that I would do anything for her, I would be the one who would hurt her the most.

My temper was explosive, and I often felt powerless in the face of it. What I hated and condemned myself for most of all was that my willpower alone wasn't enough to stop these explosive expressions of rage.

While I would never physically harm anyone, let alone a woman I loved, I now question whether she could have known that, given the intensity of my temper. At my core, I questioned whether the intermittent presence of my rage would prevent her from dropping into a sense of safety with me, and having this question run in the background of our relationship gutted me. Once the emotions quieted down, I would feel a sense of intense and visceral shame.

For the longest time, intense volatility was just a regular aspect of my romantic relationships. I didn't question it because I lacked the awareness that a different sort of relationship was even possible. It was not until I was well into my thirties that I had enough exposure to other people's relationships that my aperture began to widen to include what healthy relating could look like. I would unconsciously attract women who had emotional violence in their family history, and as a result, carried a similar imprint in her nervous system. Her rage and outbursts made it all too easy for me to avoid looking at my own issues. It was easier to just devolve into blame and accusation. I attempted to justify the patterns: We are passionate people. We fuck and fight with intensity and passion.

Then along came Sophia.

I was driving her back to the airport for her return flight to Seattle. We had made it to the airport but not yet to her drop-off point. We had gotten into a fight in the car. I slammed on the brakes and yelled at her to *get the fuck out!* I remember screaming at her. I remember the door slamming. I remember locking her out and yelling to her that she could walk the rest of the way. I can't remember the specifics of the fight. My memory of this encounter is extremely and unusually vague; however, what I do remember is that that was the last time I ever saw Sophia again.

I was shocked; I didn't understand why or how she could completely shut me out of her life after this incident. We had plans to go to Peru together. Our flights were booked, and our itinerary was planned. She cancelled it all and ceased all contact with me. She wouldn't answer my calls or respond to my texts or emails. She was just . . . gone.

I was deeply confused. I didn't understand. I was upset and angry about it, too. Mostly, though, I was hurt and bewildered by her abrupt disappearance. It took me about six months to understand that she had a boundary—and in my rage, I had crossed it. She would not be in a relationship with a man who treated her that way.

In all the other relationships I had been in thus far, instances like the airport incident were not unusual. Perhaps one of us would break up with the other, but we would always come back. Violent eruptions of rage had become so normalized that I truly could not comprehend why Sophia had left. We had just spent the past ten months in a beautiful relationship with much closeness, love, passion, and intimacy—yet all the while, the shadow of my dysfunctional anger was never far away.

It took me far longer than I would like to admit to recognize that Sophia ghosting me was an incredible gift. The stunning shock to my system forced me to realize that behavior like mine might actually not be OK, that my inflamed moments of blind rage could be terrifying to a woman—no matter how deeply passionate we were or how much I adored her.

Sophia simply would not allow herself to be the focal point for my unresolved wounds. It was many years before my propensity for volatility was removed from my system, but it was through the gift of Sophia's ghosting me that I came to realize that it doesn't matter how a woman (or anyone) treats me, I am still responsible for how I respond.

Little did I know that my most toxic relationship ever was still ahead of me. I share more about that relationship in chapter 46, "The Harmful Expressions of the Wounded Feminine." Sometimes it can take a while to move from first insight of the problem to fully learning and integrating the lessons.

Flash forward a couple more years. Once I was able to confront my anger, I was finally able to do something about it. I consciously chose to not enter a relationship again until I had a better relationship with myself first. I focused the energy I would normally place inside my drama-filled relationships on healing myself, building my business, and finding my voice and footing in the world. As I became more whole, a more whole woman showed up.

Elie and I spent the first year of our relationship on separate continents, seeing one another every couple of months, which allowed me to continue focusing on myself, my own healing, and building my business. Once Elie returned to the States and we began spending more consistent time together, those same patterns of volatility started to creep back in. This time I had the capacity to see the regressive patterns, and I searched for ways in which I could be supported to release those old, painful ways of being in the world.

Finally, I found two practitioners of a specialized trauma-release modality and found my way to working with them. I moved a lot of old, stuck energy that had been trapped in my body. After that, those hair triggers that I had had largely disappeared.

What my long, confronting journey with my relationship to my anger has taught me more than anything is that much uncontrollable anger and rage is rooted in trauma. By releasing the trauma from the body, we release the rage. It is very clear to me that we don't fully understand anger and rage—particularly the anger and rage of men. I believe that we need to acknowledge the breadth of men's trauma if we are ever going to successfully address the problems that we as a culture blame on men's anger.

It wasn't until relatively recently that I realized that anger serves a purpose and function. As I have come to understand what anger is trying to communicate, I have been able to form a better relationship with it. My anger tells me when I or someone else has crossed my boundaries.

My anger wasn't the sole problem in my relationships; it was also my inability to recognize that my partners were crossing my boundaries, usually because I failed to communicate them. Instead of recognizing and communicating that my boundaries were being violated and doing whatever was necessary to re-integrate mutual respect (including leaving the relationship if need be), I just responded with anger—and then I would condemn myself for my angry outburst.

We are only beginning to understand trauma. Our collective understanding will continue to grow rapidly, and with it there will be a corresponding rapid growth in the healing of the trauma. If we do not confront our traumas, our pain will continue to be passed down through generations.

As I have shared, I was resentful toward my dad for many years. Somewhere in my thirties, I learned that his father had been a raging alcoholic. As a result, my dad never drank. He broke that part of the family chain. With all of the anger and rage in my household growing up, it is hard for me to imagine what it would have been like if my father had been a drinker. He did, however, carry on the rage, so I saw it as my responsibility to overcome and break this part of the chain. Otherwise, I would pass it on to my own children for them to deal with—and I refuse to do that.

I made a promise to myself in my late teens that I wasn't going to have a family until I knew that I wouldn't raise them in a household like the one I grew up in. As a result of this vow, I was almost forty years old before I got married and had a baby. It took me that long to learn how to recognize and release the stranglehold trauma had on me.

Slowly, I began to accumulate lived experience that proved to me that I was no longer reflexively obedient to that place of anger and rage. I finally felt confident that I could raise a family in a peaceful, loving, and emotionally safe home. To this day, this bone-deep knowing brings me a deep sense of peace and is one of the greatest accomplishments of my life. I am only sad that it took so long—and am deeply apologetic to all the women I have loved who were on the receiving end of my once-uncontrollable rage.

> How do you relate to your own anger? What are the triggers that set you off? Do you tend toward being more hot-headed, or do you tend to stifle your anger? Who do you have in your life whom you can talk with about your relationship to anger?

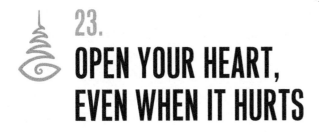

23.
OPEN YOUR HEART, EVEN WHEN IT HURTS

After a particularly harsh breakup, my desire to be a counterpoint to the pick-up artist world backfired. *I mean, look at me*, I thought. *I'm fucked up. I feel destroyed from the inside out.* My heart had closed up, and there was that part of me that began to wonder if perhaps this community that I shunned so much was right after all. Fueled by their rhetoric, I allowed my anger and resentment to heighten. I used the erotic power I had cultivated to just go fuck a lot of women without much care. This attitude was short-lived, but it was enough to show me the dangers of what happens when men shut down their hearts. If there is a time in my life on which I look back and have regrets for how I treated women and the impact I may have had on them, it is this one.

To the casual observer, my behavior may not have looked very different from how I was over the previous few years. At a deeper level however, it was quite different. It came from a different place within me, and I am sure it had quite a different effect, as well.

When I first discovered my erotic power, I went on a little spree of seducing many, many women; however, I was asking myself, *How can I leave a positive imprint on each of these women? In a world in which so many women distrust men and the masculine so much, how can I help her open once more? How can I help her heal her relationship to the masculine? How can I help her learn to trust again? How can I help her release old wounds and traumas? How can I leave her better than I found her?*

And I did just that. Many of these women are still in my life. Many of them still care very deeply for me and are deeply appreciative of the experiences we had together. The night of the wedding celebration to my wife, I realized that out of one hundred fifty attendees, more than a dozen were former lovers of mine. I view this as a positive barometer.

Contrast that to the time period during which I was "fucking away the pain." I felt hurt and empty inside. There was a bottomless black hole inside of me that I was trying to fill with sexual conquest. I began to use women to distract and anesthetize myself from my own pain. My heart was shutting down, and I swore I would never let myself be hurt like that again. *I will never allow a woman to have that kind of power over me or cause me that kind of pain again.* I could feel a hardening and numbing sensation wash over me.

Stories were going through my head, like: *This is what happens if I allow myself to trust a woman, to really open up to a woman and allow myself to love—I'm only going to be taken advantage of or betrayed.* Since I was connected to the internet, it didn't take long to find communities online who wanted to reinforce that voice within me.

I had had no idea that websites existed where men came together to commiserate in their frustration and heartbreak. Instead of acknowledging their own pain, these men instead project it outward, attaching dark, misogynistically drenched beliefs to justify their unprocessed emotions. As I read through page after page and experienced those men expressing their rage, I knew that blaming others is never the answer. However, I could feel the seductive quality to it. Misery does love camaraderie.

I could see my darkest impulses reflected in the voices and stories of other men online who were going down deep, dark rabbit holes of angry commiseration. Seeing men with so much vitriol, blame, and lack of responsibility, and allowing their rejection and heartbreak to lead to such misogynistic rage, made it clear to me that, come hell or high water, there was no fucking way I was going to give in to my pain and anger. I knew that if I allowed myself to go down that path, it would destroy me.

Despite my anguish, I made a choice that no matter how scary it might be to open my heart, it was the only way I was going to find what I really longed for. I took on the internal frame of *How can I use this painful experience of another relationship crashing apart to open my heart up further?* It is an understatement to say that it was not always easy. I knew that opening my heart meant opening up to the possibility of being hurt again, yet somewhere inside of me, I knew that allowing myself to stay in my own misery and heartbreak would never create what I wanted in my life: to love and to be loved. I knew it was the only way to experience the love that I really desired. There was no other way.

Let's be real. It is a risk. However, the choice is equally clear: either take the risk of being hurt again or guarantee never experiencing real love ever again.

What are some ways that you could risk opening your heart even further? Where are you commiserating in your pain instead of allowing yourself to open once more? What are you afraid of? Are you willing to risk pain and loss for the possibility of love?

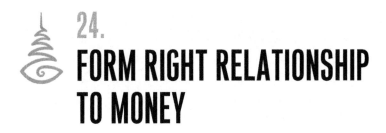

24.
FORM RIGHT RELATIONSHIP TO MONEY

As I mentioned before, I grew up in a blue-collar, working-class household. My dad was a mailman. My mom mostly didn't work. I grew up always hearing about how rich people were different from us. I was told that there were things that were for us and things that were not for us. When I moved to New York City for college, I carried these beliefs with me.

I was going to New York University on scholarship and maxing out all available loans in order to be able to live in the city. Still, that meant eating ramen noodles for lunch and two slices of pizza and a Coke for three bucks for dinner. I made an art out of finding the cheapest available options in Manhattan for everything I needed. I learned to live with certain blinders on, believing that a tiny subsection of the city (and the world) was available to me; the rest I just tried to look past, as if it weren't there.

Going to one of the most expensive universities in the country and being a working-class kid, I was very aware of the differences between me and most of my classmates. I didn't know how to connect, and just felt like I was different, and the friends I did make would want to do activities I couldn't afford, so I stayed behind.

I took this relationship to money with me beyond college. My girlfriend had gotten a full scholarship and stipend for a master's degree in botany at the University of Leiden in the Netherlands. Following my heart, I moved to Europe to be there with her. I was essentially an undocumented alien, and nobody would hire me. Sporting my freshly minted NYU degree, I felt increasingly dejected. I finally got hired off the books at a youth hostel in Amsterdam, changing bedding and cleaning toilets for the equivalent of twenty-five bucks a day.

In graduate school, as I became more politically activated, I came to identify as an anti-capitalist anarchist, taking on the belief that money was the root of all evil, so of course, if money is evil, then having money is evil. I didn't want to be evil, so I lived with relatively little money. I was focused on how little I needed to make in order to survive. This mindset kept me in a cycle of living at the poverty line throughout my twenties.

Contrast that with today. I now run a multi-six-figure business with an eye on seven. I regularly have conversations with multimillionaires—even a billionaire once—who are looking to learn from me and who are happily paying me an extraordinary amount of money for my help in creating changes in their lives through my particular area of expertise. Now there are times when I make more in a day than I used to make in a year.

What happened? Beyond all of the institutionalized obstacles and injustices that are all too real, the biggest challenges with going from a lower economic class to rising up through the class system are the internal psychological barriers. I had to reprogram much of how my psyche relates to money, resources, and how the world works. I had to shift out of a belief that there is not enough to go around and that I don't have enough and never will. I had to reprogram the internalized belief that the only way to make money is to fuck over other people. I had to reprogram the belief that having money was evil.

Step by step, I began to replace those beliefs with a belief that there is more than enough in the world, and that this is a universe of plenty. With support, I took on the belief that the resources I need—money and other forms of resource—are floating all around me, all the time. I had to reprogram my belief to one in which I could get paid for the value I provide to other people. It took work to get over my psychological hurdles, but I learned to believe that my gifts are valuable and that there are people who will joyfully trade their hard-earned money for the value I can provide to them through my gifts. I learned to take on the belief that when I approach creating money as a creative act, my inner artist could get involved and make creating money fun!

I came to believe that I could bring my value system and my integrity into how I create that money, and that the more money I make, the more resources I have to create the differences I want to create in the world. I could also use money as a tool for measurement: the more money coming in symbolizes a greater breadth and depth of impact I am having in the world.

This was a complete paradigm shift for me around how to relate to money. As I started to take on more positive frames around money, creating it became easier. Being in business for myself, I had to learn how to have direct conversations with individuals in order for them to hand over money to me—hundreds, thousands, even many tens of thousands of dollars at a time or more. Through having hundreds of these conversations, I have learned to hold my clients' own processes of moving through their money shit, each time seeing some of my own bullshit stories reflected in their words. Listening to my own internal money stories come out of the mouths of other people made it easier to see how flawed the stories were, and with that, easier to let go of.

I have now known enough people across the entire spectrum of socioeconomic classes to recognize that there are well-intentioned and ill-intentioned individuals in every stratum of society. Among the very poor are people who are self-focused and willing to fuck you over to make a buck. Among the very rich are people who are self-focused and completely willing to fuck you over in order to make a buck—and this is true in every stratum in between. Among the very poor, there are people who will give you the shirt off their back and dedicate their lives in service to others, doing everything they can to take care of their fellow human beings. And among the very richest stratum of society are people who are dedicated to using their vast resources to do everything they can to drive change and uplift their fellow human beings. Again, the same is true in every stratum between.

I look at the world, and while there is incredible beauty to be found, I also see far too much pain, suffering, and injustice. In my heart, I see a world that is possible, and I am dedicated to doing everything I can with my life to create that world, regardless of whether I will live long enough to see it or not.

I focused on how to create a relationship to business and money in such a way that I could live in integrity and in alignment with my values. I took on the belief that I could create money helping create a world I want to be living in. I chose to believe that the more money I created, the more I could invest in creating that world, a world I want to leave to my children. I believed it was possible, and I made it so.

What are your values around money? What does being in integrity with money mean to you? Is your relationship to money congruent with your principles and values? Is the way you make money congruent with your principles and values? If not, what would it look like if it were? How would you know when you had enough?

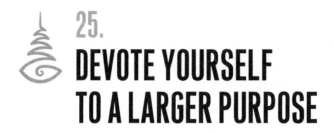

25.
DEVOTE YOURSELF TO A LARGER PURPOSE

I feel fortunate that I became connected to a strong sense of purpose at a young age, catalyzed by the tragic event of Anjali's rape, long before I had ever heard of the concept of purpose.

To commit oneself to purpose is not a little act. Purpose is not the same thing as fulfilling the white-picket-fence American dream. Purpose is a reason for existing. I believe we are all here for something far greater than simply being consumers—I believe we are here to be creators and contributors. Purpose involves committing to something larger than yourself. It is an endless stream of choices, actions, and decisions in the direction of that purpose. It can require sacrifice. It can require doing things you don't necessarily feel like doing. If you are willing to truly stand for something, and you are sincerely committed to it, then there will be times when your purpose will ask you to go far beyond what is comfortable. And it is extraordinarily fulfilling.

At this point in my career, I have created a successful company that continues to grow. I have ever-increasing impact and influence in the world around that which I call my purpose—but I didn't start this way. I started from a feeling of powerlessness as I mourned the effects of a distorted and immature masculine sexuality on Anjali's life as the survivor of teenage rape. It was in those moments that I made the decision to be part of the solution. I had relentless tenacity to move in that direction over the course of my life despite challenges, obstacles, and failures along the way—of which there were many and likely will be many more in the future. Committing to a purpose in this way builds strength, courage, character, and resilience. It requires humility and a willingness to learn from others as well as a willingness to invest in one's own growth.

David Deida speaks about the importance of a man living his purpose, and if you don't know what your purpose is, then your purpose is to find your purpose. I have mixed feelings about how this notion is expressed, because it is an incomplete, masculine, linear perspective.

In contrast to Deida's perspective, I believe that finding purpose is not always a straight line. Steve Jobs, the founder of Apple, took a calligraphy class in college just for fun. There was no intentional reason or purpose behind doing so other than it was interesting to him at the time. As a result, ten years later, he built a variety of beautiful typography into the first Macintosh computers, something completely unheard of in the world of technology at the time and that has since become standard across all platforms. We now take for granted that we have hundreds of fonts to choose from.

When you are connected to your sense of purpose, you can draw from disparate experiences and parts of your life, all of which can inform and contribute to what you are doing. Devote yourself deeply enough to your purpose, and the separation ceases: you are your purpose. Everything you have experienced in this life has contributed to creating who you are—and therefore, your purpose.

If a man hasn't found something he will die for,
he isn't fit to live.

— Martin Luther King, Jr.

At this point in my life, I am deeply rooted in my purpose. I have committed my life to evolving masculine consciousness: to examine our notions of what masculinity is, let go of the aspects that do more harm than good, and both claim and strengthen the best parts of our masculinity. I use my life as a powerful stand for men to learn to adapt to the rise in women's power, and to do so in a way that embraces and actively supports their rise. The Evolved Masculine supports the rise of women across the globe because he understands that her rise helps call him further into his own greatness, expanding his capacity and potency in the process.

I have found great value in holding a purpose that is so large that I might not be able to complete it in the remainder of my lifetime. It is much like when the great Martin Luther King Jr. spoke of having seen the promised land and understanding that "I may not get there with you."

Now that I have a daughter, I have a very real, tangible reason for my work, and because of that reason, a future I am working toward. My purpose as a man, a father, a husband, and the founder of the Evolved Masculine is to shift male culture, masculine consciousness, and the structures of our societies so that as my baby girl grows into being a young woman, she has all the freedom of expression and safety she needs to create the life of her dreams. This is my daily inspiration and what I source my purpose in—especially when life feels challenging.

Having my bold, Edenic vision gives me an always-expanding place toward which to direct my energies. I can dream, envision, and hold steadfast to this seemingly impossible future and work moment by moment toward making it so. Holding a massive vision, believing in it strongly and fully while knowing that I may not live to see it but being devoted to it anyway, gives my life purpose—just as I found the value in going huge with my vision of the Erotic Rockstar and the Evolved Masculine archetypes. Envisioning something bold enough to create that magnetic pull energy will inspire you with possibility and draw you forward even in times of difficulty or opposition.

> Where do you feel the most sensation and energy, whether it's pure, idealistic hope and optimism or rooted in pain, or fueled by anger? This can be a compass directing you toward your purpose. What do you care about? What really matters to you? What are you willing to truly devote your life in service to?

26.
FIND YOUR UNIQUE CONNECTION TO SOMETHING GREATER THAN YOURSELF

As I was her sole male descendent, my grandmother took particular steps to make sure I was raised with an understanding of Jewish history and our familial religion. Once weekly, on Saturday mornings, I went to Hebrew school, where we would have two classes: one on learning Hebrew, and the other on learning Jewish history. I began attending when I was eight years old, and at thirteen, I had my bar mitzvah commemorating my passage into being recognized as a man in the eyes of the synagogue. I really enjoyed it. I became the most committed Jew in my immediate family and would lead the sedars (ceremonial meals) during the high holy days in our home.

After my bar mitzvah, I continued my studies for another two years for the confirmation process that our synagogue offered. When I completed that at fifteen years old, I thought, *Well, now what?* I did everything my synagogue had to offer. What do I do now to further explore my faith? While I had read passages, I had never read the whole Bible, so starting with Genesis 1:1, I began. By the time I had finished Exodus, my faith was on shaky ground.

I had two major difficulties with much of what I read. One was a conflict of values. Passages that condone slavery and severe mistreatment of women really irked me. The other difficulty was that what I read conflicted with my sense of logic and reason. I would read different passages that directly contradicted one another. Maybe A could be true, or B could be true, but both A and B could not be true.

Around this time, Nine Inch Nails's album *The Downward Spiral* came out, and my friend Damien got the CD. He came over to my house and played it, and I thought, *What the fuck is this noise?* He forgot the album at my place when he left, and I ended up listening to it on repeat for the next few weeks. The third track, "Heresy," in a nod to Nietzsche, proclaims the death of God while pointing to the hypocrisies of the church. I had never heard anything like it before—such clear heresy and questioning religious ideals so directly.

I spent the next couple of years trying to figure out what to do with my now-shaken faith. *OK, so maybe the Bible is bullshit, but what about my relationship to God himself?* In college, I took classes in comparative religion, studying a number of eastern religions: Buddhism, Taoism, Hinduism, Confucianism. I found a lot that I really liked but still kept running across the misogyny.

I started to identify as an agnostic-leaning atheist. I didn't know if there was a god or not, but probably not. I held this view for ten years. Then, like many people, I had a crisis of faith. It was clear that the structures of religions and the way they were taught were stuffy and stale. They had lost their magic and were rooted in rote traditions.

I was a non-believer until I was twenty-six years old. After being arrested for the third time in just over a year for political-activism-related work, and after spending three days in jail at the shit end of police brutality—both my rotator cuffs were torn and my cervical disc herniated—I went on a downward spiral of my own. I descended into what I can only describe as a psychological and emotional breakdown. I lost my faith in humanity. The world was going to hell in a handbasket, and nobody seemed to give a fuck.

I hit a point at which I could see only darkness in the world. If somebody said to me, "It's such a beautiful day. The sun is shining, and the sky is blue," I would find some way to twist it and point out all that was wrong. Truth was, I couldn't see the beauty in the world anymore. Quite honestly, if I had kept going the direction I was headed, I probably would have ended up in jail or dead within a couple of years. (A former lover's boyfriend was shot and killed at a protest in Guadalajara. The incident made the cover of *Rolling Stone* magazine. When I read his story, it was easy to see how it could have been me.)

I could see how extremists are made. When things seem hopeless, it can feel like drastic measures need to be taken just to wake people the fuck up. My mind went to some very dark and destructive places, as I had fantasies of just burning shit to the ground. Thankfully, something shook up inside of me, and I realized that if I took that step, there would be no turning back.

I had a crush on a Mexican revolutionary anarchist woman I had met at the Free Trade Area of the Americas protests in Miami the previous year and who lived in Mexico City. She invited me to come down and travel through southern Mexico together. I had just seen *The Motorcycle Diaries*, about Che Guevara's journey leading up to his becoming a revolutionary leader and icon, so the idea sounded particularly romantic to me. Besides, I had nothing else to do. My friends couldn't deal with me anymore, so I threw a backpack on my back, and with two hundred fifty bucks to my name, I headed down to Mexico, figuring I would find a way to spend the next couple of months there.

Unfortunately, two people spinning downward do not lift each other up. While we had some fun, we fought a lot, and things weren't working. (She did help arrange for me to spend a week in a Zapatista Mexican revolutionaries' village. I was interviewed by three black-ski-mask-wearing, large-gun-toting, intimidating men. They discussed the situation in Spanish—which I only minimally understood—as they decided whether or not to accept me into their village for the week. They did, but I nervously wondered whether I was going to get out of the room alive—but that is a story for another time.)

After the revolutionary village adventure, I split with my anarchist lover, packed up my things, and headed for Palenque, a rumored backpackers' paradise. There are many stories from my time there, but suffice it to say that a couple of days in, I had what I can only describe as the start of my spiritual awakening. I had hit a point in my life where the only thing I knew anymore was that I didn't know anything, and I simply gave up. Whatever I was holding on to, I just let go. It is hard to put into words, but whatever I was clinging to—this notion that I had it all figured out, that I knew what was going on in the world, my sense of self-importance in it all—I gave up. I just let go.

I can point to a single day during which everything changed, when a switch flipped, and every person I met, every conversation I had, allowed for this shift within me to occur.

At this little enclave of globetrotting adventurers, I met all these people who viewed and experienced the world through a very different lens than I did.

They held a much more optimistic viewpoint—they believed that the world was waking up, that an evolution of consciousness was occurring. This was 2004, two years before Facebook was invented. I had no social media connections to such things. I didn't know that there was even such a thing as a conscious community, and quite honestly, if I did, I would have just made fun of it. But in the emotional state I was in, I let it in.

Within a couple of days, I stumbled across a middle-aged Mexican couple who sat with me at length and listened. They could feel the anguish in my heart and my utter confusion toward life. They had such calmness about them, and an acceptance of me and where I was at. They told me that in two weeks they would be leading a week-long Toltec initiation and invited me to be a part of it. In this initiation, I had a series of experiences that defied my sense of reality. I ultimately came out of it with a clear sense that there was more to this universe than I understood. Not only was I now open to it, but from that point forward, I would begin actively seeking out and welcoming a deeper understanding of the ineffable.

This is the point at which I consider myself having intentionally stepped onto a spiritual path. I believe that we are all walking a spiritual path; it is just a question of how aware we are of it. Like anything else, when you bring greater awareness and consciousness to walking your path, your experience changes. You often learn and grow more rapidly in that direction and with greater ease. But a spiritual path is not all light. It is not all easy. It can be extraordinarily difficult and present harrowing challenges.

I had to learn to connect to something larger than myself. Just because the religion I grew up in and the Christian church that was all around me were not ideas I resonated with didn't meant that there wasn't something deeper to be found. Religion and spirituality are not the same thing. Spiritual experiences come in many forms. They can happen when you least expect them, and perhaps, if you aren't paying close attention, you may not even realize the magnitude of what has transpired. The Evolved Masculine must find his connection to something larger than himself. His connection to others, this planet, and the universe itself is unique to him. The more intentionally this relationship and connection are consciously cultivated, the greater they will serve you in your own life.

What religion or spirituality did you grow up with? What is your relationship to those beliefs today? Have you found your own unique connection and relationship to your spirituality? If so, what has become possible for you since forming this personal spiritual connection? If not, what do you imagine it looking like if you did?

PART 3
SEXUAL SELF-MASTERY

27.
FROM PREMATURE EJACULATION TO MALE MULTIPLE ORGASMS

I have worked with thousands of men, and the vast majority of them want more and better sex. They want to be the best lovers their women have ever had. They hunger for a deep sense of confidence in themselves and in how they engage with women. It is important to them to feel like they have control over their bodies instead of simply being at the whim of their bodies.

I had sex for the first time when I was sixteen. Predictably, my first couple of times were, let's say, rather brief. I was with my first love, Jeanette, for over a year, and thankfully, I had the opportunity to practice and improve. I remember one particular sexual interlude in which Jeanette was on top of me, riding me. I watched her go into some sort of orgasmic, out-of-space orbit. She was just writhing her whole body and trembling. Her eyes rolled back in her head, and she screamed out loud with wave after wave of orgasmic bliss rolling through her body.

I remember looking up at her, feeling detached and completely disconnected from the intensity of her experience. She was in an apparent state of ecstasy that was completely foreign to me. I didn't know what the hell she was experiencing, but I knew that I had never felt anything like that before—and I wanted to.

After witnessing Jeanette enter such an ecstatic state of sexual pleasure, I set off on a quest to understand and experience similar states of pleasure in my own body. To my dismay, everything I found essentially stated, "Sorry, dude, you're out of luck. Men can come more easily than women, but women who find their connection to their sexuality and orgasm have worlds of pleasure available to them that simply isn't available to men."

I didn't like this story.

A couple of years later, I came across the book *The Multi-Orgasmic Man* by Mantak Chia and Douglas Abrams. I thought I had struck gold. *Yes! This is what I'm talking about!* I started reading the book but couldn't connect to it at all. As a Chinese Taoist, Mantak Chia places a particular focus on conserving sexual energy "for health and longevity." Suffice it to say that at nineteen years old, I still thought I was invincible and had no care about such things. I was interested in discovering new heights of pleasure and becoming the best lover ever. The book had complicated diagrams of a man in a chair imagining energetic circuits in his body, and all I could think was, *What are you talking about?* I put the book on a shelf and forgot about it for years. Despite my rebellious nature (or maybe because of it!), eight years later, I ended up finding my own innovative way to becoming multi-orgasmic.

After much experimentation, I realized I was regularly having experiences in my body that most men didn't even realize were possible. Word spread about my newfound "abilities," and a guy I knew in my community asked me to teach him to be multi-orgasmic. I explained that I didn't know if that was possible and questioned its teachability, but fortunately for both of us, he insisted.

We got on the phone once a week. I would ask him questions, and based on his responses, I would give him different pieces of customized guidance based on what I understood from my own experience. Within a few short weeks, he was lasting longer in bed than he ever had before, and six weeks after that, he had his first non-ejaculatory orgasm. This was steadfastly followed by another such orgasm, and then another. Within two months of that first call, he experienced his first multiple orgasms. He went on to describe our work together as some of the most important and impactful work he had ever done in his life. The process of evolving from being at the effect of his own biological response to learning how to have mastery over his sexual expression gave him a renewed sense of confidence, both in himself and as a sexual being. He stood straighter as he walked through the world.

In light of the impact our work had for this man, I began to give the work more intentional attention. I reverse engineered what I had been exploring and created my first online video training program, then called *Orgasmic Mastery: From Premature Ejaculation to Male Multiple Orgasms*. Over the course of twelve weeks, I brought men step by step through the process of learning the practices, tools, and techniques they needed to master in order to unlock these new sexual possibilities.

Over time, and by immersing myself in teaching men about their own sexuality, I came to understand that before a man can begin to explore his multi-orgasmic potential, he must first learn to have control over and choice about when or even if he ejaculates.

As dozens and then hundreds of men went through my programs, I asked more questions and began to see patterns in their experiences, their frustrations, and their desires. I came to understand that men who were struggling around ejaculatory control were often in deep emotional anguish. There is a massive industry that sells men pills, creams, numbing products, and fear-based, superficial courses promising to help them overcome premature ejaculation. Personally, I believe that most of it is bunk—simply a manipulation of men's pain points and insecurities to make a buck.

Through interviewing my customers and clients, I was exposed to a powerful cross section of the lived experience of men across the globe. I went deep into the esoteric realms: tantra, sacred sexuality, technical Taoist energetic practices, and even canonized Western academic approaches to sexuality. Essentially, I distilled thousands of years of esoteric practices, stripping them down to tangible tools that men could put into practice in order to experience real results in their own bodies.

I discovered the precise pain points and wounds that men hold that get in the way of their erotic growth. I learned firsthand how important having a level of mastery and control over his body and sexual impulses is to a man's confidence and personal power.

It was not uncommon for me to work with men—even highly successful CEOs and multi-millionaires—who from the outside looked like they had it all. They had checked off the box of building incredible material success in their lives while ignoring and running away from a dirty little secret they had—until they hit a point sometime in their mid-thirties, forties, or even fifties where they couldn't ignore it any longer. The dirty little secret? The pain, dissatisfaction, and shame of not having control over their own bodies, not feeling like they could satisfy a woman or experience real satisfaction themselves. For many men, it had become an obsessive concern. The pain and shame had become so acute that they couldn't focus on anything else anymore. They had to solve the problem once and for all.

Sexual self-mastery serves all men, far beyond ejaculatory issues. Ejaculatory choice is what I refer to as the first of four gates of sexual self-mastery. Once you have walked through this gate, whole new worlds of erotic possibility open up for both you and your lover. The second gate is the ability to experience full-body orgasms, in contrast to orgasms that happen primarily in your groin. The third gate involves learning to separate orgasm (the peak flood of pleasure through your body) from ejaculation (the release of fluid from your body), and with that, opening up your ability to experience non-ejaculatory orgasms. Passing through the fourth and final gate allows you access to the holy grail of male multiple orgasms— and yes, not only are they a real thing, but with both commitment and attention, they are possible for you!

Sexual self-mastery involves building a strong sense of connection to your sexual energy as an *energy*, and then learning how to work with this energy, play with it, and channel it by choice. Sexual energy is powerful life force energy itself. It is literally that which creates life. You don't need to relate to your sexuality as simply a distraction from the rest of your life; it can be a potent energy that you can learn to channel into creating what you want with your life.

Sex is powerful. Sex can transform you and your lover. But first, you must get into right relationship with it. It doesn't start with her, it starts with *your connection to yourself.*

While I will continue to weave in personal stories to give you a sense of my own path of attaining sexual self-mastery, this section is a bit more technical. I would like to remind you again that to maximize the results in your own life, you need to do more than read about these various tools and techniques. Sexual self-mastery comes only through embodied practice.

As I explored my ego of the Erotic Rockstar, I formed a unique connection to my sexuality that was reflected back to me time and again as being extremely different from what women normally experience with a man. That difference helped make my sexual encounters feel intensely magnetic and safe while still carrying a perceived edge. Through accepting and embracing the wholeness of my sexuality, I gave my lover permission to be a fully expressed sexual being herself.

Learning to release any shame and judgment around my sexuality made it easy for me to accept and embrace her sexuality without judgment. This is a powerful gift, as most people are walking around carrying shame, fear, guilt, and judgment about their own sexuality. Rather than owning our feelings about sex, we often unconsciously project onto others, making them wrong for the negative feelings we carry about ourselves.

This path of sexual self-mastery will lead you to both confront and release any culturally induced baggage of shame, guilt, and fear you still hold around your sexuality. You will replace that baggage with an embracing of your sexuality as part of the whole of who you are, and integrate it into your being: mind, body, and spirit. Your sexual desire is not about needing, grasping, or taking anything from anyone, and so you are challenged to freely own your sexuality and desire—not for conquering or taking, but rather, to be a powerful gift to share.

> How would you describe your relationship to your own sexuality? What were the messages that you received about sex growing up? How will you experience life differently by attaining sexual self-mastery?

28.
WE DON'T UNDERSTAND MALE SEXUALITY

We don't understand male sexuality. What we don't know, we fear, and in many ways condemn and shame. As we transition from boyhood into manhood, as this powerful sexual energy starts to come online, we aren't given very good guidance around what to do with it.

The truth is, your sexual energy is extremely powerful. It can be used for good or evil. Your cock can be a weapon that can do harm, and it can be a "wand of light"—a *lingam*, as it is referred to in Sanskrit. Your sex is a powerful force that can be a gift to enliven and help a woman open, surrendering to the fullness of her being and to life itself.

There are ways in which she can touch into this life force energy on her own through self-pleasure. There are ways in which her sexual energy is hers, and she can access it on her own. There are also ways that she can access the transformative nature of this energy only through you. A man can take a woman deeper than she can take herself. Unfortunately, a lot of women's sexual experiences with men do not measure up to this ideal. In fact, there are many women who have better orgasms on their own than they do with a man and whose erotic experiences with men are mostly disappointing. Just about every woman has had encounters with men that were very disappointing. Sadly, those are the lucky ones, as there are still many more whose negative experiences with men extend far beyond disappointment and into the traumatic.

Her disappointment can come from one of two directions: either you simply don't care or you simply don't know. You don't really care about what is going on in her body, what she is really feeling, wanting, needing, or desiring because you're too busy focused on yourself, your own dick, or your ego; or you might care, but you don't know any better. Too often, your ego is in the way of your taking the steps required to learn.

Here's the deal: For you to understand her sexuality, you need to start by truly understanding your own sexuality and by radically understanding your own body and how it works. You need to learn to connect to the subtle sensations that your body can experience. As you learn to connect to your own body, your own sexuality, and your own pleasure in new ways, you will then naturally, easefully bring this new way of connecting to her body, as well.

Masculine Sexuality Has Been Contorted

Everything we have been taught about masculinity and male culture limits men from experiencing the truth of their sexuality. What we have been taught about ourselves actually diminishes our capacity to learn the fullness of our sexual expression. Male sexual culture has had a strong conquest basis—getting another notch on your belt—which is not about feeling at all. Rather, this conquest focus is a mental construct more than anything; it is also likely why there is never enough.

You can never get enough of what you don't need, because what you don't need won't satisfy you.

— Dallin H. Oaks

Much of what we have been taught about what it means to be a man actually keeps us further away from our true sexual expression and possibility. "Man up." "Toughen up." "Feel less." "Man, you're just too sensitive!" All of this conditioning teaches us to disconnect from our bodies. Disconnecting from what we feel in our bodies makes us more impervious to pain, yes, but also more impervious to pleasure. Quite simply, our social conditioning has made us numb, and it is not possible to be both numb and an extraordinary lover.

Masculine Sensitivity Has Been Distorted

Everything men have been taught about themselves actually distances them from their own sexuality. Consider the example of premature ejaculation. The existing narrative and cultural meme about PE is: "Oh, you're too sensitive."

No. This is dead wrong. If you are coming more quickly than you would like, this is because you aren't sensitive *enough*. Instead of learning how to cultivate your own sensitivity, you have been made numb by the pervasive cultural myths and messaging to men. Because you have not yet cultivated enough sensitivity, there are things happening in your body that you are completely unaware of, and so you go into habituated patterns that cascade into ejaculations that seem to just happen to you.

(Note that erectile dysfunction and premature ejaculation, while occupying opposite ends of the spectrum, are symptoms of the same root problem: lack of sensitivity.)

Masculine sensitivity is a powerful taboo in our conquest-driven male culture. Male sensitivity—the antidote to many of the problems that exist in the realm of human sexuality—is brought into the conversation only when it is distorted and tied to issues like premature ejaculation. This is a massive stranglehold on the true, healing function of male sexuality, and is perpetuated by profound misunderstandings of how our bodies function.

Most of the discoveries and realms of possibility laid out here in Part III require you to completely break out of the "man box." This requires you to get present and learn to truly and fully inhabit your body and your feelings. You will be challenged to increase your sensitivity and learn how to feel subtlety. In return, you will experience heights of pleasure and fulfillment beyond anything you have ever known.

How well do you know your own sexuality, really? Take a moment to think about how your childhood, teenage, and adult conditioning has dulled your ability to feel both pain and pleasure. Are there ways in which you are aware of your own untapped sexual expression? Are you willing to unwind old imprints of male sexuality that may be incomplete or distorted? Do you feel a desire to do what it takes to know who you are as a sexual being, free from societal conditioning?

29.
THE CRUELEST CUT: CIRCUMCISION

If ever you wanted proof that we don't understand and in fact fear male sexuality, look no further than how widespread male circumcision is in the United States. Circumcision rates peaked in the 1970s (when I was born) at roughly 90 percent. Today, those statistics are closer to 55 percent, yet still, the majority of boys born in the United States have a scalpel taken to their penises shortly after being born to have the most sensitive part of their genitals amputated—without having any ability to consent to it.

An infant boy, in a state of human innocence, has an iodine solution rubbed onto his genitals (often causing his first erection outside of his mother's womb), which is then met with a scalpel. In other words, his first sexual experience is one of violence and violation. As if simply by the nature of being born male, our industrialized medical system takes a "corrective action"—directly implying that there is something inherently and essentially wrong with male babies. The act of circumcision communicates that there is something defective that needs to be fixed.

The medical establishment in the United States adopted circumcision in the late 1800s as a method intended to stop young boys from masturbating. Over the years, as that reasoning was eventually rejected, new "justifications" have been invented to continue this insane practice, yet to this day, circumcision is still an essential way in which our society goes about desensitizing—and dehumanizing—male human beings.

I was circumcised at eight days old in a Jewish *brit milah* ritual. For the next twenty-three years, I never thought twice about it. After graduating from New York University, I moved to San Francisco, where I went through a seventy-five-hour training to be a certified sex educator through San Francisco Sex Information (SFSI), an organization that provides free sex information. After certification, I volunteered to work for SFSI's hotline, which meant that I spent evenings twice a week in their office answering phone calls (yes, on a landline).

People would call in to have their anonymous questions and concerns about anything sexuality-related answered nonjudgmentally.

One evening between calls, I was going through the bookshelf and saw *The Joy of Uncircumcising!* by Jim Bigelow, PhD. I'm sorry, *what?!* It appealed to my always-curious inner sexuality psychonaut, so I picked it up and started thumbing through it.

The first half of the book is dedicated to the history of circumcision as well as its physiology and anatomy. The book describes the inner lining of the foreskin as being developmentally similar to the inner lips of a woman's vulva. Just as her inner labia are made of mucous membrane tissue meant to stay protected, warmer, pinker, and more moist than external skin tissue, so is the glans (the anatomical name for the head of the penis) and the inner part of the foreskin. The second half of the book focuses on a subject that was equally startling to me: *uncircumcising,* or what is generally referred to as *foreskin restoration.* Bigalow details a series of methods that a man can use to essentially regrow his foreskin. I was repelled and transfixed, all at the same time. I didn't know what to think of it, but I was intrigued.

With promises of greater sensitivity, healing, and better sex, I thought, *hmmm . . . I'm not so sure, but hell, an experiment having to do with my dick?! I'm in!*

I took the book home with me and cautiously proceeded with my first experiment. I pulled my cock out from the hole in my boxers and began examining it. With my newfound knowledge, I noticed something I had never taken note of before: a little more than an inch back from the head there was a very obvious thick, brown scar line that went completely around my shaft. *Oh, shit, that's from my circumcision! How did I get to be twenty-three years old and never even think about this mark that's inscribed into my own genitals?!*

The book suggested pulling forward any loose skin and using a Band-Aid to tape it up over the head. Obstacle #1: I didn't have any loose skin to work with. I would later learn that circumcisions can vary quite a bit based on the aesthetic preference of the person doing it (isn't that just a bit fucked up itself?). The *mohel* (the person who performs the Jewish rite of circumcision) who performed the excision on me cut me quite tight, so instead, I pushed the glans back in toward my body, pushing more of the shaft tissue into the pelvic cavity, and taped the skin forward with the Band-Aid.

As you can imagine, it was a bit uncomfortable at first, but for the purpose of the experiment, I committed to keeping it taped forward like this as much as I could, twenty-four hours a day for one full week, removing it only to pee and shower (I had no sexual partner at that time). It was a minor pain in the ass, but I kept my commitment, and at the end of the week examined myself closely to see if there was anything to all the fuss.

I was shocked by what I observed after only seven days. All of the mucous membrane tissue, meaning both the head of the cock and the tissue that is forward of the circumcision scar line, was much more sensitive, pinker, and had a light moisture to it! *What? That's crazy! How is that even possible?*

Then something else really baked my noodle. For at least the previous five years, I had cracked skin on the left-hand side of the ridge of the head that never got any better. Granted, it probably never healed in part because I was masturbating so frequently, but it was also because it was exposed and dried out all the time. It was always irritated, and I had to be careful when I masturbated or it would become very painful (not that it stopped me). Well, after this short seven-day experiment, the cracked skin had healed to the point that it was barely noticeable!

Frankly, I was shocked. I was skeptical about this method to begin with, but these tangible changes after such a short time threw me into a tailspin. I continued to restore my foreskin off and on over the next couple of years. I found the process to be difficult, especially when I was in a sexual relationship. I never got more than halfway through the process, but even with the half-assed attempt I made, the changes to my sexual function were remarkable. Most notably, whereas previously the skin had been painfully taut when my penis was erect, now the shaft skin has a mobility to it, gliding up and down over the erectile tissue beneath it.

Clearly there was something to this foreskin restoration thing. *And if there is something to the restoration part, then maybe there is something to having a foreskin in the first place—in which case, what am I missing out on?*

I had what is known in the anti-circumcision, or *intactivist*, community as the famed "obsessive epiphany." With the realization that there was more to this whole circumcision issue than I had been led to believe, I became obsessed with learning everything I could possibly find about the subject.

Over the next couple of years, I read more than twenty books on circumcision as well as every scientific study I could find. Unfortunately, it was a case of "the more you know, the worse it is." Here is a brief synopsis of just some of the rarely discussed impacts of circumcision: More than twenty thousand fine-touch nerve endings are permanently removed; there is a keratinization (callousing) of the remaining mucosal tissue and head, leading to loss of sexual sensation, especially as men become older; there is a complete change in how the sex organ functions; and perhaps most insidiously, it is now understood that traumatic injuries impact us for the rest of our lives because they physiologically change the human brain. This is true even if we cannot consciously recall the original incident.

Confronting my own circumcision injury as well as deepening into the socio-ethical landscape surrounding this highly controversial policy often consumed me. I remember one particular instance in which I had spent the entire day deep in circumcision research. When my girlfriend came over all horny and ready to go, she playfully reached down and pulled out my cock. I looked down and was suddenly overcome with immobilizing grief about what had been done to my body without my consent. I froze, feeling a tsunami of emotions that had been stored in my body since I was an eight-day old infant. Not only could I not proceed with what would have been a steamy, erotic encounter with my girlfriend, but I was also unable to fully express what I was feeling—what my body was remembering and releasing.

Looking down at my nakedness, all I could see was the giant scar that was left on my penis, the phantom limb of the amputated foreskin that I will never know, and the echo of the wound that was inflicted on me without my ability to dissent to a procedure that would permanently affect me: my sex, the neurology of my brain, and literally, my life. In those moments, I understood that I had crossed a threshold; the needle had moved from this exploration being an intellectual curiosity to one that was having a deeply intimate and emotional impact on me.

Over the next couple of years, as I deepened into the reckoning phase of my circumcision, I experienced a lot of intense emotions. I felt violated. I felt deeply traumatized about something that the larger society said I should be grateful for. I felt sadness and grief about the fact that I would never be able to experience my genitals and sex the way nature designed them. I felt anger and rage toward my parents for believing that they had the right to make this choice for my body. I felt animosity toward my religion for continuing this traumatic blood ritual over many thousands of years. I lost trust in the once-sacrosanct medical community for violating their Hippocratic Oath of "First, do no harm." I felt rage and confusion toward American society at large for remaining in denial about what should be so fucking obvious: *men are not born defective and in need of being surgically "fixed!"* I became increasingly disillusioned. *How the fuck can we be doing this and normalizing it? Why is it not even being talked about?*

Now, more than fifteen years later, I have largely moved through these emotions, yet even as I write this, I am aware of a certain grief inside of me that I have simply learned how to live with.

In retrospect, I don't think it was an accident that I began to walk this path of sexual self-mastery sometime after my exposure to the circumcision issue. Part of what released me from the pervasive feelings of disempowerment and depression that I experienced when I confronted my own grief and anger about circumcision was bringing my attention to what is possible for me to experience with my body and sexuality. (This is a huge part of what the teachings in this book are based on: you are going to grow in the direction that you place your focus.) As long as I was focusing on the detrimental impact of circumcision, I was creating a life in which I was disempowered, angry, and grief-stricken.

After many years of integration, I was able to acknowledge the very real harms that have been done and bring my focused attention to what is possible for me to experience sexually with this body of mine exactly as it is. This focus led me down a path that allowed me to have experiences in my body that—circumcised or not—most men don't realize are possible, let alone are experiencing themselves.

The Reckoning

I believe that an aspect of mastery in any realm involves realism: seeing things as they are. Men must acknowledge the impact of having been circumcised without getting stuck in the state that "there's something wrong with me now, and I'm irreparably harmed."

The other reason to become present to it—to allow yourself to acknowledge the harm of circumcision—is so that you don't perpetuate it. The biggest reason why circumcision continues to be performed is because we pass it down from generation to generation; circumcised fathers circumcise sons. "Well, I was circumcised and I'm fine, so it'll be fine for my son."

On a deeper psychological level, I have come to believe that the circumcised man perpetuates circumcision because if he did not circumcise his son, he would need to confront his repressed feelings about his own circumcision. Instead, he rationalizes, *My parents would never harm me, I am not harmed, and I would never harm my son, therefore, circumcision must not be harmful, so of course I will circumcise my son.* If the circumcised man did keep his son intact, he would have to acknowledge and confront the fact that he himself is missing something from his own genital anatomy.

Furthermore, the perpetuation of circumcision feeds on the cultural distortion that men aren't supposed to be victims. We aren't supposed to complain or express that there is something wrong or that we are feeling pain. A man can't complain without being told to quit his complaining, often with cliché shaming: "Man up. Just suck it up and deal with it."

There hasn't been room for the ways in which men have also been victims of some of the cruel programming of our patriarchal society and the ways that they, too, have been harmed.

Circumcision isn't sexy. It is not easy to talk about, and it is often met with extreme resistance or shutdown in both men and women. Mothers and fathers are often grief-stricken when they learn of the potential harm they unknowingly subjected their baby to, and men who have been circumcised as infants do not want to meet the grief and rage that remains held in their bodies. But the hard reality we *all* must come to terms with is that we are all complicit, both men and women, in perpetuating an act of violence upon tiny little baby boys.

When a foreskin is cut away from a penis, it sends a physiological shockwave through the penis—the point of the most densely clustered nerve endings on the male body—and then directly through the spinal cord and into the brain stem. In this moment, the brain of an infant boy becomes permanently ed.

I am not for a single second condoning bad behavior by men nor using circumcision as an excuse to justify a single drop of the blood that drips from the hands of some men in our culture—but I *am* saying that we must all be willing to pull back the veil on the ways we have been programmed and conditioned to normalize a "consensus reality" agreement that is causing harm to infant boys who, yes, then grow up to be men who hold positions of leadership and power in our world.

My own reckoning with my circumcision has been one of the most painful and liberating aspects of fully owning my sex and my power as a man. Sexual self-mastery is indeed confronting as fuck. The dragons to be slain are inside of us, so we must be willing to look them squarely in the eye before we can stand boldly in our own power as sexually free men.

> Had you ever thought about circumcision before reading this chapter? What thoughts and emotions did this bring up in you? If you are circumcised, you may feel anything from grief and anger to numbness, or even a mixture of all three. Know that you are not alone, and by committing to the path laid out in the remainder of Part III, you can still begin to expand your sexual pleasure and capacity now and throughout your life ahead.

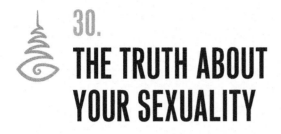

30.
THE TRUTH ABOUT YOUR SEXUALITY

I want you to know that your sexuality is your birthright. It is powerful. It is not something you need to be ashamed of or have any guilty feelings about. It is something that you can embrace and celebrate. Despite the clear warnings from the #metoo movement, masculine sexuality does not need to be harmful or destructive. It can be enlivening, life-giving, empowering, and transformational for both you and whoever you are sexually engaging with.

It is not your fault if you didn't know these things. Chances are you have received extremely subpar education and training around your sexuality. Your sexuality is infinitely complex, and one of its gifts is that you can actively, consciously explore it throughout your entire life. Your sexuality is good, and it can be a force for good. The more you release any culturally induced sexual shame, guilt, and fear, the cleaner your sexual expression will be, the more attractive you will be, and the greater a gift your sexuality will be to others.

Women are sexual creatures, and their innate, natural sexual expression can look quite different from yours—but there is a beautiful gift in that, as well. As you both have an opportunity to share your sexual expression with one another, you get to learn, understand, and have a whole new world of sexual expression introduced to you through her, just as she gets to have that experience through you.

The problem through much of history has been that men have focused on pushing their way of sexual expression onto women and forced them to contort into expressing themselves based on a male fantasy of what their sexuality is supposed to be. In this new era that is unfolding, with women owning and claiming their sexuality and desires and discovering their own sexual power in new ways, that is no longer going to fly. You can have your fantasies fulfilled and still create the space for her authentic feminine sexual expression to unfold and blossom. It truly is a beautiful thing to behold.

Reimagining male sexuality is not about limiting your sexuality or losing anything—at least, it doesn't have to be. It can be what I call "expanding your palette of pleasurable possibilities." A safe and turned-on woman can be a sexual powerhouse and can take you to places you never knew were possible. As she continues to explore and understand her sexual possibilities on a larger level, there is an opportunity for you to rise up and do so, as well. As she begins or continues to expand and deepen her understanding of her own sex, there is an opportunity for you to do the same—and in fact, she *wants* you to do the same so that you can truly meet her. Only in this way can you both be on this path of exploration and discovery together.

I want you to know that there is such a thing as healthy masculine sexual expression and that sexual self-mastery is a foundational part of it. I want you to understand your sexual energy. I want you to understand your body and allow sex and pleasure to inspire you enough to cultivate presence, embodiment, and your ability to really feel—including subtle sensations—because the rewards are the most obvious and delicious in sex. But they also affect every area of your life. As you become a more whole man, you become a more free man.

Your sex is a core part of you as a man. It is not something that needs to be relegated to the shadows or compartmentalized by locking yourself in a room, pulling out the porn, and furtively masturbating to get off so you can then tamp your sexuality back down and move on with your day. Nor does your sexuality need to be relegated to weekends at bars and clubs with a clear, focused agenda to release the pressure valve by getting laid.

Your sexuality is much larger than that. You can spend your entire life exploring your sexuality, and there will always be more to explore. I want you to know that by committing to the path of sexual self-mastery, you will come to know your sex as a gateway to some of the most profound experiences of your life and as a powerful energy that you can tap to fuel your greatest dreams and visions.

Do you value your sexuality? Do you respect, appreciate, and honor it, or do you hold it in shame? Do you feel fulfilled in your sexuality? What do you imagine a sexually empowered man to be like? Most importantly, who do you imagine yourself to be as a more fully sexually empowered man?

31.
WHY SEXUAL SELF-MASTERY MATTERS

Sexual self-mastery is the foundation of life mastery. When a man attains true ejaculatory choice (the first gate of sexual self-mastery), the world changes for him. Something in his system relaxes.

If you are like most men, you want to feel at cause in life rather than at the effect of life. You want to feel like you have control of your destiny and your finances and that you have choice in the woman you are with instead of feeling like you are just settling for whatever comes your way. You want to feel like you have choice and control of your body instead of simply being at the whim of whatever your body does to you. In short, you want to feel at empowered choice in all of life—and your own body is the foundation of that.

We don't get any education and training around sexual self-mastery, ejaculatory choice, or how to navigate this powerful sexual energy inside of us, so we either think we have to repress our sexual energy because it is not acceptable or that it is in control and running the show. Sexual self-mastery is the door to a better, more potent way of expressing your sexuality.

Many men do find their way to modulating the intensity of their sexual energy and lasting longer—and many don't. They develop patterns in their bodies, neurology, and unconscious energetic patterns that drive them toward rapid ejaculation. Men who deal with this as an issue suffer tremendously from it; hence, there is much money to be made in the field. Too many unscrupulous individuals and businesses are happy to make a buck, selling the man snake oil because they know he is desperate.

What I found through working with so many men all over the world is that when a man feels like he doesn't have control in this area of his life, it can come to affect all aspects of his life. It can leave him in a state of disempowerment that bleeds over into everything he does. It can cause him to feel like less of a man.

When a man feels like less of a man, he is not able to live into the fullness of who he is capable of being—and honestly, a man who feels like less of a man can be a dangerous man, as he often feels like he has something to prove. Far too many harms have been done in this world by men who were trying to prove to the world, to other men, and to themselves that they are "real men."

Conversely, when a man does have sexual self-mastery and walks through that first gate of ejaculatory choice, he gains a certain swagger to his step and walks with his head held a little higher. He has a deep sense of confidence in his being, as he is relaxed knowing that he doesn't have any fear or concern when it comes to his sex. Having true ejaculatory choice and mastery of his sexuality changes how he shows up in the sexual interaction. He shifts the energetic pattern away from the constant driving force of ejaculation and toward coming fully into the present moment-to-moment play.

He is able to hold and contain his sexual energy. It can flow freely without restriction and move through his entire body, allowing him to last as long as he wants and to feel more pleasure throughout his entire body. Something completely changes for her and her sexual experience, too. When she knows that he can last as long as he likes, she doesn't feel like she has to be chasing her orgasm, trying to make sure she comes before his ticking time bomb blows. When she can relax, she has the ability to soften more fully into her feminine, to surrender more fully into her body and all of the pleasure that she is capable of experiencing, which opens her up to whole new levels of orgasmic possibility.

The things he learns and integrates into his body in order to have sexual self-mastery changes how he experiences his body, sex, women, and the world. In order to have true ejaculatory choice, experience full-body orgasms, non-ejaculatory orgasms, and multiple orgasms, a man must learn to be in his body and to truly feel deeply.

Too many men have instead learned to tighten down, numb themselves, and plough through life. You will soldier on and get through it, but you will miss out on so much joy, connection, and sensation—and so much of life. Likewise, you can do like so many men do and learn to last longer by numbing out, by dissociating from your body and feeling less so that you can do what you believe is expected of you and last long enough to satisfy her.

However, there is an native path forward. You can learn to feel and attune to energetic subtleties, to be present to the moment-by-moment reality of what is happening in your body. By bringing awareness into your felt sense and deepening into subtle sensation, you can notice and attune to what is happening for the woman you are engaging with. Opening to feel changes the game. It is no longer just a mental game of trying to figure out what to do and what she wants—now you can *feel* it. Your body becomes the tool to feel what is going on for her. If you can't feel what is happening inside of you, you won't be able to feel what is happening inside of her. When you can feel it, you can sense into her and respond moment by moment—which unlocks whole new worlds of sexual possibilities.

Does this mean that you can't ever have porn-style hardcore jackhammer fucking? No, it doesn't mean that. However, as you expand the number of colors in your palette of pleasurable possibilities, your paintings are going to look different, and your sex is going to look—and feel—very different. The "red" of that fast-paced driving force toward the orgasm becomes but a single color in a vast spectrum of possible erotic tones.

A man with sexual self-mastery is self-sourced. He is in connection with life-force energy itself. When a man shows up from a place of fullness, with his sexuality as a gift he has to offer, instead of showing up from lack, where sex is something he needs and has to get out of her, the energetic dynamic is completely different. It is far more potent and enjoyable for everyone involved.

Mastering your sexual energy means being in control of it instead of being controlled by it. We have an axiom in the culture about men having two heads and only enough blood to flow into one at a time. Mastering your sexual energy means being able to equally choose yes or choose no. Pussy can be waved in front of your face, and you can choose: no, this is not really what is going to be best for me or for her. And you can choose: yes, this will serve both of us.

Alongside the axiom, there is messaging in our culture that says if sex is available to a man, he has an unspoken obligation to go for it. Further, if sex is available, his not going for it is a sign of weakness or that something is wrong with him, that he is less of a man. *What are you, gay?* This is distorted, archaic messaging that needs to be updated. Your power comes from your ability to discern who or what you say yes to and who or what you say no to. This goes for sex and every other area of your life, as well.

If you want to feel truly empowered sexually with women, you must master your own sexual energy. Women are accustomed to being the sexual gatekeepers. The expectation is that a man will always want to have sex with her, so she decides if and when—and he should just consider himself lucky. *Fuck luck.* You can learn to draw out and entice her desire, but only by mastering your own. The more you expand your capacity to hold sexual energy and sensation in your body, the more you can spark and help amplify her sexual desire. (We explore this in depth in Part IV, "Understanding Women and the Feminine.")

Walking the path of sexual self-mastery has completely transformed how I experience sex in more ways than I could have anticipated. Letting go of the notion that the only way to make her come is to go harder, faster, more, I learned instead to tune in to her sexual energy and what her desire is really asking for in that moment. As I developed my sensory acuity, I was able to tap into the waves of sexual pleasure as they built, not only in my own body but inside of hers, as well. Once I learned to feel those subtleties, I was able to intentionally direct the building of her next peak as well as to ride wave after wave of pleasure with my lover without fear of wiping out.

A man with true ejaculatory choice can last literally as long as he wants to. He consciously chooses whether he wants to have a two-minute quickie; twenty minutes of hot sex; two hours of marathon sex; or go two days, two weeks, two months, or even two years without ejaculating. It sounds like an exaggeration, but with true ejaculatory choice, time is irrelevant.

Once a man learns how to take his sexual energy as it is being generated in his groin, his cock, and his balls and spread it throughout his entire body, he diffuses the ticking time bomb of ejaculation. As this energy generates, it spreads throughout his body. He learns different ways of releasing it through and from his body instead of just out the tip of his cock with ejaculation. With that ability to move and disperse his sexual energy at will, he is no longer a slave to his need to come, and there is no risk of unintentionally blowing.

The false programming we have been sold is that if you don't ejaculate, you are going to be uncomfortable or even in pain. That does not need to be true: you can learn to enjoy running sexual energy in your body without a needed final moment. This is not to say that you can't ejaculate. Ejaculatory orgasms can be incredible, and quite frankly, through this process, you can learn to experience the most powerful ejaculatory orgasms of your life. But the key is to learn to have ejaculatory choice so that you can choose whether to ejaculate or not. You can choose when to. You can choose if to. And you can find incredible fulfillment in any of those choices.

Everything changes when a man has sexual self-mastery.

> Do you find yourself worrying about whether you are going to come too soon or not at all? Does this stress keep you from enjoying sex and being present with your lover? Does it result in coming before you want to, thus feeding the cycle? If so, next time try focusing on being present with your lover and all the feelings that are happening throughout your body.

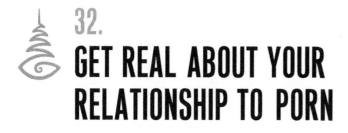

32.
GET REAL ABOUT YOUR RELATIONSHIP TO PORN

My first introduction to sex and sexual feelings was through porn. I was probably no more than five or six years old. We would visit my grandparents' house, and my grandfather had a stash of porn magazines in a little stand next to the toilet. Suddenly, I was spending a lot of time in the bathroom. I would look forward to going to my grandparents' house, in no small part because I knew I could look at more of those pictures of naked women. It was many years before I made any connection between my fascination with looking at those nude, erotically charged images of women and masturbation.

When I was eleven years old, I went to get the bathroom scale out from underneath the sink in my parents' bathroom. Hidden in the back was a VHS tape of what turned out to be adult video previews. I was thrilled, as I had only ever seen still pictures in magazines. I waited until both my parents were out of the house, excitedly put the tape into the VCR, and sat enthralled, consuming the five- and six-minute clips marketing new adult films that were being released.

In the videos, I not only saw women having sex, I saw naked, sexually aroused men for the first time, as well—men with gigantic cocks that seemed to have little in common with my own. I saw the man aggressively ramming into the woman, only to pull out and stroke his cock until white fluid spewed out the tip, often landing on the woman's sweaty body. *Whoa!* Within moments, I was stroking my penis for the first time.

Lo and behold, I can produce that fluid, too!

And so the connection between masturbation and porn began for me—at the age of eleven, more than five years before ever having sex for the first time.

When I finally did start having sex, what really had me in awe was that I experienced sex as better and more profound than what I had imagined from what I had seen. What porn didn't prepare me for were the feelings of deep intimacy, connection, and vulnerability I experienced. I felt loved and accepted in a way that I had never known. That was profound.

Today the climate is quite different in that we now have access to limitless internet porn. Anyone anywhere can get their hands on more pornography than they could consume in several lifetimes. It is difficult for me to imagine how much porn I would have been exposed to during my teenage years if I had had that kind of unadulterated access.

People speak sometimes about how porn establishes unrealistic expectations for what sex is and looks like, but I don't think that that is the real problem. When we speak of porn in that way, it further glorifies the porn experience. Don't get me wrong, I have had extremely hot "pornified" sex, and I have had sexual experiences that looked nothing like porn and were far more profound and powerful for me and the woman I was with, so it isn't just that porn sets unrealistic expectations for sex; it is that it can put us on a path of chasing after a type of sex that isn't even necessarily going to fulfill that deeper yearning within us. And yet, due to the injection of porn into our homes and the ways it has saturated so much of male culture, men can spend their entire lives chasing after that porn ideal—and miss much of the fulfillment that is available to them in real-life sex and intimacy.

When men measure themselves against a porn ideal, and if they are not experiencing the satisfaction they believe they are "supposed to" or that they believe they are seeing on screen, they internalize harmful narratives: "I'm not enough of a man," "My dick isn't big enough," "My penis doesn't get hard enough," "I'm not lasting long enough (or fucking her intensely enough)," or "Maybe I am not aggressive enough." In other words, when a man compares his sexual experiences to the film-set porn ideals he has been consuming since he was a boy, the story he internalizes is, "I am simply not enough."

Deep insecurities can—and often do—set in from an early age. Some part of him is trying to make his sexual experiences look more like the sex he sees on screen in the hope of arriving at a state of fulfillment he secretly longs for—

even though it can only be found once he stops trying to replicate what he sees in porn.

The entire porn industry is ripe for disruption. We need new models—including onscreen models—of sex that show us what is truly possible to experience through sex. We need to be exposed to models of total mind-body-spirit sexual connection and the transcendent aspects of sex, the potency of deep presence and what that can open up. Have you ever even seen a man in deep ecstasy, riding wave after wave of full-body, multiple orgasms along with the woman, in porn? Probably not. Why not? Well, maybe there are a lot of things that the porn industry doesn't know about sex. There is a lot more available and possible for you.

Porn is generally designed to rapidly excite the man's sexual circuitry, so it can be difficult for him to slow down enough to appreciate and value those subtler sensations and what he can experience only through slowing down. Most porn is through a particular old-paradigm male fantasy lens that rewards a fast-paced race through required linear foreplay, only to arrive at a frenzied jackhammering penetration so that the man can get off: kiss, kiss, lick, lick, suck, suck, fuck fuck, come. Man comes. Sex is over. Done.

From a young age, men see these women (porn actors) onscreen having crazy, screaming orgasms from men being sexually aggressive with them in a particular style. Naturally, they assume, *Oh, I guess that's what women must really like.* Human beings learn through mimicry, so when we are repeatedly exposed to images, both still and especially moving images, our brains are literally being wired to imitate these images and scenes.

Porn infiltrates the image banks of sex in men's minds, and then, naturally, they go into real life and attempt to reproduce what they saw. Women are also exposed to porn and have also internalized, *Oh, that's what men must really like.* She then tries to contort herself into these behaviors and enactments to try to please him. As a direct result of porn, literally no one, neither man nor woman, gets to experience their own authentic process of sexual discovery. Instead, they both try to perform an *idea* of what they think they are supposed to be and do.

I have had a very large number of sexual partners and experiences. The vast majority of my sexual experiences have been positive—most of them extremely positive. I have experienced women having every conceivable form of orgasm: multiple orgasms, blended orgasms, anal orgasms, squirting orgasms, and more. I have been with multiple women whose first orgasm with a man was with me. I have been with women who exclaimed to me in many different ways how they were experiencing the most powerful orgasms they had ever had, within the best sexual experiences of their lives. I have had women tell me that they felt addicted to sex with me—and even still, I have held insecurities about the size of my cock.

Where do you think this insidious voice comes from? I spent hours and hours (and hours) in my life consuming on-screen sexual imagery where the average cock size is eight inches. Seven-inch cocks are actually on the smaller end of the cock lengths featured in porn. Despite all the ways I should—and do—know better, these insecurities could still affect me. Through a combination of sexuality workshops, sex parties, and other environments, I have had the privilege of seeing a large number of naked (even aroused) people in real life, both women and men, that showcased a reality very different from on-screen porn. Still, the size of my own cock can fuck with my head. I can only imagine the negative impact of the porn mega-cocks on men who don't have the experience of receiving so much positive sexual feedback. (This, of course, excludes those readers who do have mega-cocks . . .)

I have noticed that there are different ways in which I can be sexual with a woman, and one is heavily influenced by the porn model. This expression of my sex is much more linearly oriented, much more focused on trying to get her to come, much more focused on my own ejaculation. This aspect of my sex is more mechanical and technique-driven.

There is another aspect of my sex that is moment-to-moment present, playful, can go anywhere in any direction at any time, and allows both of us to run sexual energy through the circuitry of our bodies and our connection together instead of simply chasing orgasms. In this space, it becomes about discovering the pleasure and bliss in each moment and deepening our state of connection and intimacy with one another. Now, to be transparent, I can find pleasure in both of these routes, but I know which one brings me my greatest, most rewarding experiences—and it is not the one that has been most influenced by porn.

We can convince ourselves all we want that porn doesn't affect us—but it does. All of my research, trainings, and teachings around neuro-linguistic programming and advanced applied psychology have helped me to understand the way the mind works and the irrefutable interconnection between the conscious and the unconscious mind. All psychological lineages confirm that when we are in a heightened state, the veil between the conscious and the unconscious mind thins, and the unconscious mind is the most susceptible to suggestion. When we are consuming porn, we are in a heightened state of arousal—and this is precisely when the psyche is most susceptible to imagery. What are you suggesting to your unconscious mind? And is it really in service to what you truly desire?

This is not an anti-porn tirade. I don't believe that onscreen footage of two or more people having sex together is inherently problematic. I do believe that the porn industry could use some serious evolution and that most men (and I include myself) have or have had unhealthy relationships to porn. In many ways, the way porn functions is similar to a drug.

I am challenging you to be courageous and look your own porn habit squarely in the eye. It is my belief that men must do this with one another by talking about it and defusing the stranglehold of shame that traps so many men. To reiterate, it is not my intention to make porn wrong, but I am taking a stand for you to be in empowered, conscious relationship to your porn use.

What is your relationship to porn like? Take a moment to critically examine your sexual behaviors and think about whether some (if not many) of your moves are inspired by professional porn actors, who are often not very connected to their authentic sexuality and are instead just performing for the camera. Are you modeling your intimate experiences with others from what you have seen on screen? If so, is that working for you?

33.

ESTABLISH A PRACTICE OF EROTIC SELF-EXPLORATION

For your sexuality to be received as a gift, there is some reprogramming to be done. The path of sexual self-mastery is about discovering something more within your sexuality than simply your orgasm or the ego gratification of notching your belt with another sexual conquest, or even of making her come (this was the trap I was in). Sexual self-mastery is about far more than simply jacking off; it begins by cultivating an erotic relationship with yourself.

I use the phrase "erotic self-exploration" (ESE) to differentiate between your typical masturbation habits and a more expansive deep dive into your own sexuality. Nearly every man masturbates; however, most men masturbate in the same way they did when they were adolescents. When an adolescent boy initially starts masturbating, usually right around the time puberty sets in, he often develops a habit of doing so as quickly and quietly as possible so as not to get caught. This is important to realize because it shows us that right from the get-go he is establishing in his system that his sexuality, pleasure, and turn-on are inherently shameful. Over the years, this pattern of furtive, goal-oriented, "efficient" masturbation sets in.

In 2006, when I was in a three-hundred-hour training to become a California state-certified sexological bodyworker, I was given a series of homework assignments that included intentional self-pleasuring. I was to bring attention to staying present in my body, paying attention to every touch I was doing, every sensation I was experiencing, and the kicker—*no porn*. I was shocked and, truthfully, humiliated, horrified, and aghast at how tremendously difficult I found it. Here I was, twenty-eight years old, and I had become so dependent on porn that the idea of masturbating without watching strangers fucking on a screen was unfathomable to me.

I quickly discovered that it was difficult for me to get aroused and maintain an erection without highly sensationalized visual and auditory stimulation. Without porn, I noticed that my mind wandered a lot. I found myself either wanting to give up on the assignment altogether or cheating by watching "just a little bit." When our addiction drives us into our cravings, addiction and recovery communities call this *jonesing*, and I realized that was exactly what was happening for me: I was jonesing for porn, hard.

This was a huge wake-up call for me. The idea that I had outsourced my own body's innate capacity to create and experience pleasure to strangers on a screen was yet another point of intense reckoning for me. Despite wanting to cheat, and despite being confronted by intense cravings, I developed the inner fortitude to turn off the porn, and slowly learned to turn on my own body.

I traced my history of masturbation back to when I first started touching myself in my early teen years. I recalled that while I definitely enjoyed porn when I could get my hands on it, I also masturbated a lot without any visual stimulation. I would enjoy touching myself simply from the state of being in awe of the process of discovering my body and the pleasure it was capable of providing.

I now became wildly curious: what had happened to me over the years? My curiosity was not just about my experience of confronting my own porn dependency. As I looked more deeply into the collective male experience, it became eminently clear to me that porn addiction was rampant and had wound its tentacles tightly around the masculine psyche and the male experience.

With my famous (among people who know me) persistence and dedication, I continued with the assignments of porn-free masturbation, and to my amazement (and relief!), over the coming weeks, finding my arousal and my pleasure on my own became easier. I found that staying present in my body, without my mind jumping out, hungry for external stimulation, became easier. I began to access new states of pleasure that I hadn't known before.

This practice created a forced intervention in my masturbation habits that was deeply liberating. It allowed me to actively explore my own sexuality in a way that I hadn't since I was an adolescent boy. This is congruent with what I see in male sexuality: men adopt a certain way of masturbating when they are in puberty that includes a rushed, secretive, shame-encoded quality. If porn had not been part of their initial experiences, it soon becomes part of the habit, so what was established as young boys becomes frozen in time *and* in the nervous system, and often never evolves further.

I expanded this assignment from my early days of sexological bodywork into the practice of erotic self-exploration, which will be the foundation on which you will walk your path of sexual self-mastery. I have been asked many times if a man can do this work when single and without a partner to practice with. The truth is, it is often easier to learn and practice when alone—it is sexual *self-* mastery. Bringing your attention to exploring your own body, understanding your own sexuality, and doing these practices without having someone else to worry about makes dropping fully into the process easier. This way, when you are next with a lover, you will have a new, incredible sexual connection with self to share with them. These practices work wonderfully in partnership, as well. That said, even if you are in partnership, for a predetermined window of time, commit to making the erotic self-exploration practice your primary focus.

Most people's masturbation habits are highly goal-oriented. Frankly, it is about getting off and coming, oftentimes quickly so you can get back to what you were doing. You are feeling stressed or agitated or are surfing the internet when up pops an image of a sexy woman. Next thing you know, you go right into that unconscious pattern, click over to a porn site, whip it out, get off, and then think, *Wait, what was I doing right before this?* and continue on with the day.

Most often, an unconscious habit or pattern arises. Something triggers the masturbation habit pattern, and you just go into it. Maybe it is anxiety in the body, a discomfort that you have learned to deal with by knocking one out so you can go on with your life. Or maybe it is rubbing one out as a way to unwind before going to sleep. Masturbation becomes a tranquilizer or a way to self-soothe a jagged and overburdened nervous system. There is nothing wrong with using masturbation as the occasional pressure-release valve. However, if this is the crux of your sexual experience, do you think perhaps it may be a bit limiting? And do you think perhaps if this is a frequent occurrence on your own that it is having an impact on your experiences when you are connecting sexually with a lover?

Your practice of erotic self-exploration is distinct from your masturbation habits in that ESE doesn't have the focused goal of orgasm—not that the goal is to not come. Rather, if there is a goal, it is simply to explore. It is to know yourself more. It is finding out what else is possible to discover with your body and sexuality. It is a moment-to-moment exploration instead of an endpoint to get to. Slow down, play, and explore—each time you do, you will find more.

If there is one major rule about what to do during your ESEs, it is this: don't fall into the routine of your existing masturbation habits. If your masturbation habit usually looks like you sitting in your chair or on your bed with the laptop open, a porn site up, and your dick in your hand, going up, down, up, down, while clicking around until you come, then your ESE can look like anything but that. Try something different that is screen-free. Open up some adventurous possibilities to explore your turn-on. How many of those factors I just described can you take out of the equation, and what can you do instead?

ESEs are about taking time with the screen turned off and being present with yourself, your body, and the sensations that are alive for you in this primal experience. This can be challenging when you are just getting started with this new practice, because you can overthink it: *I'm not experiencing turn-on the way that I'm used to. I'm concerned that I am not going to get turned on just by my own body.*

As long as you are doing anything but your typical habits, you are expanding your sexual experience. If you have a porn-reliant masturbation habit, then starting this exploration may hold challenges. You may find that it is difficult for you to get or stay hard when you are not staring at and hearing heavy stimulation. When in the space of an ESE, it does not matter if you stay hard. This practice is not about going from soft to hard to harder to hardest and then to climax. It is about just being with the truth of your moment-to-moment experience. It is masturbation as meditation.

Masturbation habits are often pretty unconscious, as though we go away and check out during it. With your ESEs, aim for the opposite state of awareness: How conscious and present can you be? How much can you stay in your body? It is about getting out of that outward focus of attention, getting out of your head, and giving yourself full permission to experience what you are feeling in your body in the moment. I promise you this: any woman you are sexual with will appreciate your learning to be this present in your body during sex and finding the pleasure and enjoyment that can only be found through deep presence.

Waking Up the Full Body

Your entire body has the capacity to experience pleasure. By stimulating your body regularly throughout the sexual experience, you teach your neurology to spread all of that energy through the body during orgasm, as well.

Neurons that fire together, wire together.

— Donald Hebb

Shift your awareness from your pelvis as the container for your sexual energy to your entire body as the container. It is a much larger container; it can hold far more. This both lengthens the time you can spend in sexual stimulation and makes it so that when peak orgasm occurs, there is far more sexual energy to explode. Just knowing this can change things instantly.

One of the practices that I have my clients do is what we call *waking up the body*. A lot of men today spend all their time in front of a screen, whether a laptop, phone, tablet, or TV. They spend much of their time up in their heads looking out, increasingly disconnected from their bodies.

One great way to train yourself to get back into your body is to start your ESEs with self-massage. Set an intention to touch and stimulate every millimeter of your body, as if you were waking up every nerve ending of your body.

Women have a tendency to already want this level of attention given to their bodies, and yet most women don't expect it from men because it is such a rare experience. Training yourself to bring your attention to stimulating every square inch of her body (by starting with your own) will set you apart from 99 percent of the men out there and make you the best lover she has ever had.

What are your masturbation habits usually like? How much do you actively explore your solo sexuality versus simply doing the same thing every time? Do you find it difficult or easy to arouse yourself without porn or fantasy? Commit to a practice of erotic self-exploration

34.
STRENGTHEN YOUR SEX MUSCLES

If you want to gain true ejaculatory choice and even experience non-ejaculatory orgasms, Kegel exercises are key. Kegel exercises are designed to strengthen your pelvic floor muscles—referred to as the *PC muscles*—the pubococcygeus muscles—or sometimes simply the *sex muscles*. These are muscles that go from your pubic bone down around the base of your cock, including your anal sphincter, and connect to your tailbone, or coccyx; hence, pubococcygeus— PC. Like any muscle, they take time to strengthen, so now is as good a time as any to get started.

I was nineteen years old when I first learned about the PC muscles. I read that the easiest way to locate them is to stop the flow of urine when you are mid-stream. The muscles you use to stop the flow are some of the same muscles that are responsible for ejaculation. I remember that when I would go into a public restroom with a line of urinals, if I was alone, I would start and stop peeing in each urinal, going down the line into each and every one, just because I could. I later learned that while this is a great way to initially identify the PC muscles, it isn't healthy to continue to interrupt the flow of urine all the time, as it can confuse the body as to when the bladder is actually empty, which can lead to infection. (And nobody wants that.)

Once you are able to feel and identify the PC muscles through stopping the flow of urine, you can strengthen them in other ways. Right this moment you can feel into those muscles and just give them a squeeze. If you find it difficult, you can also push your middle and ring fingers up into the area known as the perineum (some people call it the *taint*)—that area between your balls and your anus. Simply press up into that area and squeeze the muscles that are beneath your fingers. You can feel them harden or create resistance against your fingers; that is when you know you have it.

Practice twenty-five quick squeeze-release repetitions with your PC muscles on a daily basis. As that gets easier, you can move to two sets daily and work your way up to fifty or even a hundred quick squeezes. Add in slow squeezes: count to five as you squeeze in, hold for five seconds, and slowly release for five seconds. Lastly, practice "reverse" Kegels, where you push out, or bear down, and then relax. They will help you learn to not tighten the muscles and be able to let go and release tension in your PC muscles at will.

35.
AN INTRODUCTION TO THE FOUR TOOLS FOR MASTERING YOUR SEXUAL ENERGY

There are four primary tools you can use to connect to, cultivate, and channel sexual energy: breath, sound, movement, and visualization. Each of these tools can be endlessly explored, and they organically support one another. Diving deeper into one will help you get more out of the other three, and vice versa. Remember, this is a path of sexual self-mastery; it is a never-ending path. This is not "Three Quick Tricks You Can Do Tonight to Completely Transform Your Sex Life Forever." These are practices to take on and build relationships with over time. They are tools you can play with and hone every time you are sexual, whether with a partner or by yourself. I would like to reiterate that most men experience their breakthroughs faster when they put their primary emphasis on learning this through their solo practice of ESE, and then bringing them in with a partner.

If the material is unfamiliar to you, then I suggest that after reading about a specific tool, go and practice with it, and allow it to metabolize in your body. Once you arrive at a place of competence with that particular practice, move on to the next chapter, and layer that tool into your practice. Reading through the material all at once and trying to work with all of the tools at the same time will be overwhelming, and then you will not take in any of the tools as deeply. Though it may seem counterintuitive, you will likely get further faster by taking your time, learning one tool at a time. To use a martial arts metaphor, when you show up for your first lesson, they don't immediately show you every move that exists.

---

*I fear not the man who has practiced 10,000 kicks once,
but I fear the man who has practiced one kick 10,000 times.*

— Bruce Lee

Practice each tool. Integrate one at a time into your body. Build a relationship with it. Find the pleasure in it.

One objection a man will sometimes have is that he doesn't want to feel like he is being taken out of the moment because he is thinking, *I need to check my breath. I need to pay attention to my sound. What is the movement I should be doing? How am I visualizing?* And now he is stuck up in his head, which is the opposite of what he needs to be doing.

It is for this reason that I suggest starting with one tool—like how Bruce Lee drills that kick again and again in practice so that when he gets in the fight, he doesn't have to think about it, his body just knows what to do. Use your erotic self-explorations as your dojo, and practice each tool. Explore your breath. Explore your sound. Explore your movement. Explore your visualization. Explore each tool until it is in your body, where you don't have to think about it, you just know it. Then layer in the next tool.

Each of these tools will help to further unlock your connection to your primal self and freer animal expression. This in turn will open up more possibilities for you, but you will initially be required to go slower and be more attentive with your movements and how they affect your overall arousal levels. Through practice and repetition you will be able to hold greater and greater levels of sensation, intensity, and pleasure in your body. Focus on these tools, step by step, and you will be well on your way to sexual self-mastery.

36.
BREATH: YOUR NEW DRUG OF CHOICE

It was 2003. I was twenty-seven years old and still a relatively new transplant to San Francisco from New York City and thus still carried with me a lot of cynicism and proverbial sharp edges. I had enrolled in a Swedish massage training as a means to support myself while I was going to graduate school. It was a two-week, one-hundred-hour intensive. I remember showing up that first day and discovering that we were going to be spending our first two days doing "breathwork" . . . and I was pissed! I remember thinking, *Wait a second. I just paid how much money? And we're going to spend two days breathing. Seriously? Two days breathing?!*

I was livid. I think the instructors didn't quite know what to do with me, but let's just say that by the end of that first day, I was converted. Once more, I experienced things in my body that I did not realize were possible. Through bringing conscious attention to my breath and learning to breathe in particular ways, I was guided, along with everybody else in the class, into what I can only call an ecstatic experience. A flood of pleasure throughout my body followed by an experience of peace, similar to having a really good orgasm—that is what I experienced from "just" breathing. The feeling had a flavor different from what I had ever known before. Understanding that our male bodies have an innate capacity for pleasure far beyond what we have been conditioned to believe was a pivotal moment for me.

Given my propensity as a sexual "mad scientist," I rushed off to see what would happen when I combined this newly discovered breath-driven pleasure with sexual turn-on. In the name of research, I cozied up to one of my female classmates (and fellow "sexplorer") so we could find out what would happen when we merged the two, breath and sexual pleasure. Being eager students, we met up outside of class that night and took turns going down on one another while simultaneously implementing these new breathing patterns, which intentionally heightened the amount of oxygen flowing through our bodies while layering in sexual pleasure. The oxygen-rich state of my body caused all the nerve endings to be activated—so much so that when she finally tipped me over into orgasm, the neural pathways throughout my entire system were lit up like the Christmas tree at Rockefeller Center.

Breath as Lover

There is a phrase in tantra about finding the bliss in every moment. When I first heard this, I thought, *Fuck you! Find the bliss in every moment . . . you know what? Some moments suck. They're painful; they're sad; they're hard. Fuck you and your new-agey, tantric, find-the-bliss-in-every-moment bullshit.*

And then, much to the chagrin of my inner grumpy New Yorker, I actually did fall in love with my breath. I discovered that I could find the bliss—a real and deep enjoyment and pleasure—in the simple act of breathing in and breathing out. And I realized the obvious: that my breath is with me all the time. If I can find bliss in my inhalation—the feeling of that life force energy filling my system—and in my exhalation, the relaxation and letting go, then that bliss is automatically available to me in all moments, no matter the situation, if I choose it. *Bliss is available to me in every moment, in every breath? Holy shit.*

I fell in love with my breath that weekend. I started to form a relationship with my breath as I would a lover. I realized that this was a relationship I could cultivate over time and that could give me great pleasure. I could treat it consciously or unconsciously, but it was only through giving it my conscious energy and attention that my relationship with my breath became a source of fulfillment for me. It was during this experience that I coined the phrase "breath as lover." Your breath is a relationship you will have throughout your entire life. Life begins with that first gasp of air, that first inhalation, followed quickly by a baby's first cry, and life ends with its last dying breath, that final exhalation. For every moment in between your first and last breath, you are breathing—it is just a question of how conscious your relationship to your breath is.

You Probably Suck at Breathing

I came to understand that most people breathe poorly. One of the reasons why my first and early breathwork experiences were so profound for me was because I had habituated an under-oxygenated state in my body. My system had become so accustomed to getting by on a sub-optimal level of oxygen that when I suddenly flooded it with oxygen, it felt euphoric. I had learned to breathe enough for surviving, though not necessarily enough to truly thrive.

In our world, it makes sense that the majority of humans do not breathe properly. Shallow breathing decreases what you feel, and when people are scared, they often hold their breath. Why? It lessens what they are feeling. There are certainly times where a situation can feel overwhelming or "too much."

We learn and rely on defense mechanisms like shallow breathing to deal with situations beyond what we can handle at the moment. These are often coping mechanisms that we learned in childhood as a means of self-protection, but we are not taught about these things. Somatic responses happen unconsciously until they are ingrained in the body, at which point they often become habits that are used in unhelpful situations moving forward, and often throughout a person's life. This is precisely the case with both shallow breathing and the tendency to hold the breath. Holding your breath is like freezing yourself. The problem with this suspension, or frozen effect, is that the trauma itself ends up getting frozen into the body.

Breath—and specifically, relearning how to breathe—can reopen those places that were shut down many years ago, the places where old, stagnant emotions, including fear and pain, are stored. Learning to open up the body through breath (and the other three tools of sound, movement, and visualization) can be uncomfortable. These energetic tools and processes can bring up emotion that you don't understand, and if you don't have the framework to understand that this is a normal response to liberating old, stuck emotion, it can cause you to shut down and not want to go there again. If it brings up stuff you aren't prepared for, it could cause you to unconsciously avoid the work and not follow through on the practices.

Most people start exploring this work because it sounds like a fun, pleasurable path to being an awesome lover. But then, *Oh shit, I was not expecting this emotionally confronting stuff.* Let me be clear: deepening into breathwork and the other three tools does mean a certain degree of emotional confrontation, but as with all hero's journeys, on the other side of the discomfort lies greater freedom and power.

What I learned from staying the course with breathwork is that we can rehabituate our system so that our unconscious breathing habits are naturally fuller, even when we aren't actively paying attention to the breath. Fuller breathing naturally leads to experiencing more pleasure in the body—in sex and in life.

Breath as Life Force – Another Day in Paradise

As long as you are alive, you are breathing. Your breath is your life force. That is fact, no matter what, but most people take it for granted unless there is an issue and their breathing is compromised. However, you have the ability to have a conscious relationship to your breath, to witness it, to become aware of it, and to it at will and notice the effects it has.

My breath practice became an exploration. Each day, hour by hour and then moment by moment, I was actively seeking pleasure in my breath. In easy situations, when I was calm and not actively doing anything, I would consciously slow down to find pleasure in my breath. When out and about, I would intentionally play a game of finding my pleasure in my breath. If I was standing in line waiting to check out at a register, I would find my pleasure in my breath. When I was in a challenging situation, I would remind myself to pause, drop in, bring my attention and awareness into my body, and once again, find my pleasure in my breath.

Breath became my solace: a little sliver of paradise away from whatever was going on in the external world. I noticed that by bringing my awareness to my breath and touching into this subtle bliss state, I could handle whatever circumstance life was throwing at me much easier and better. I began to understand that I was building the capacity at the level of my nervous system to allow for relaxation, presence, and pleasure—simply by consciously harnessing my breath and allowing my nervous system to regulate.

Breath and Better Sex

As I started to consciously explore my breath, sex became a completely new experience. Through the process of slowing down and deepening both my inhalations and exhalations, I learned to break the habit of tensing up in the presence of pleasure, and eventually trained my system to relax into the pleasure. I learned to open and widen into the pleasure instead of constricting the sensations of pleasure in my groin.

This constriction happens when our breathing becomes rapid or we hold it, and the body tenses. Sexually speaking, when we hold our breath, we are concentrating and locking up the sexual energy into a smaller space—in this case, in the pelvis. But sexual energy has to move, so when we lock it down in that way, it is going to move the one way it knows how, which is out the tip of the cock in ejaculation.

Instead of concentrating the energy in the pelvis and your cock and balls in anticipation of ejaculation, the practice becomes: slow down; deepen your breath with long, cooling breaths to relax the body; and allow the sexual energy, the pleasure, and the intense sensation to move through the whole nervous system. Through intentional use of your breath, you can begin to develop the energetic mastery to modulate your arousal levels, surf the waves of sensation and pleasure, and expand the sexual energy throughout your body. The result of this expansion of sexual energy out of the pelvis and into the full body leads directly to the experience of feeling more present in your entire body and lasting longer.

I began to ask myself, *How do different ways of breathing affect what I feel during sex? How do they affect my sexual response, my level of arousal, and the way I experience pleasure?* Through this consistent practice, I have learned that I can use my breath as a means to intentionally shift my energetic and feeling states to modulate my arousal levels and surf the waves of sexual pleasure without fear of wiping out.

If you are like many men, as you become increasingly aroused, your breathing automatically becomes more rapid, and you may even start to hold your breath. These ways of breathing are highly effective if you want to ejaculate, because that is precisely what they will make you do. If instead you begin to slow down and deepen your breath, you will relax the musculature of the body, particularly as you exhale. Those slow, deep breaths will support you in dropping into your body, feeling more grounded, and relaxing into the present moment. Those long, cooling breaths will allow you to regulate your nervous system during sex so that it is not being overloaded too quickly and leading to ejaculation. This technique alone may do wonders for helping you feel more in control over when you come.

Expanding Your Capacity

How slow can you take your breath? How deep can you take it? Whatever you think I mean by that, I probably mean slower and deeper still. Explore your capacity to take the deepest breath you have ever taken in your life. How deep is that? At the height of your breath, take a sharp inhale and expand just a bit further. How much can you elongate your exhale and draw it out? How empty can you go? When you are completely empty, force out one last push, and then see if your next breath can be even deeper than that and your exhale even more empty.

What we are doing here is expanding your capacity to hold energy as well as growing your ability to completely release and empty out any old, stagnant energy you are carrying. One of the major reasons why a man ejaculates quickly is because his nervous system is uncomfortable holding pleasure and sensation in it. Once it surpasses its capacity, it releases out through ejaculation, returning the body to homeostasis. Use your breath to expand your capacity of what you can hold in your system through this game of expanding your breath capacity. This will also stretch your system to be able to take fuller breaths with greater ease.

Breath beyond the Bedroom

I have learned that how I breathe affects how I feel. When I am calm, I breathe in a deep, relaxed way. When I am angry, my breath feels like hot smoke blasting out of my nostrils. When I am sad, my breath becomes shallow and staccato. When I am in ecstasy, I use my breath to expand and prolong the sensation of pleasure and orgasm.

When my wife gets really upset, whether through sadness and tears or her own anger, dropping into my breath—just slowing it down and deepening it—helps me maintain my energetic sovereignty and not get swirled up in what she is experiencing, while still being present with and loving toward her. It is easier to maintain my open heart without feeling like I need to defend and protect myself.

I learned to explore. *How deep a breath can I take? How slow can I take it?* I created a little game for myself. *Can I make it slower still? And deeper still? Can I make it slower still? And deeper still?* I did this until I learned to inhale in such a way that I look like I am not even breathing, as I am drawing it out so long. Learning to work with my breath in this way has helped me to quiet my mind.

As soon as I go into these slow, deep breathing patterns, all of the mental chatter of my mind gets a little quieter. As I use this tool more and more, I can even create stillness in my mind, which helps me be more present with my partner and more clear and focused with my work. It helps me be more magnetic and charismatic to others and to know that I can handle whatever life throws at me. Using this foundational tool, I stopped being reactive, and now I can respond from a place of calm and clear-mindedness.

Falling in love with my breath has had consequences far beyond sexual self-mastery and ejaculatory choice. Breath is the foundation of life. Through the practice of bringing awareness to and building a relationship with my breath, I now use it to help me be more grounded as I walk through life and as a way to regulate my nervous system. My breath has become a way for me to calm myself and to deal with my emotions. If I become triggered and feel angry, I can use the practice of slowing down, deepening my breath, and focusing on my exhale as a way to re-find my center. Conscious breathing is a profound resource for men as they potentiate their expression in the bedroom—and beyond.

Breath is the foundational tool upon which the other three sexual self-mastery tools are built. The more conscious and aware you are of your breath, the more present you will be in your life. By cultivating intimacy with your breath, you will become increasingly grounded and at ease in your body. You will notice that life's intensity becomes a challenge instead of a struggle. I have done a full 180 in my relationship to my breath—from a cynical New Yorker to a devotee of breath—and all aspects of my life have exponentially improved as a result of deepening into this conscious practice. Everything from my sex to my bank account has been positively impacted by the simple act of filling my lungs and diaphragm with an abundance of oxygen and life force energy.

All this from the simple act of breathing in . . . and breathing out . . .

What are your breathing habits? Do you notice that you can take deeper inhalations and longer exhalations? Try to consciously do so. The next time you are intimate with yourself or a partner, instead of stressing about ejaculation or whether you are going to make her come, try being intentional with your breath. Do you notice a difference? Apply this intentional breathing to other situations that create stress in your life, beyond your sexuality. Do you notice similar improvements in your performance and ability to cope with stress?

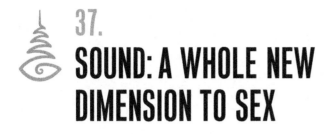

37.
SOUND: A WHOLE NEW DIMENSION TO SEX

Of the four self-mastery tools, sound came in last for me. It was also the one I found to be the most confronting. It is a harsh truth of American culture that porn is the primary place where most people get to see other people having sex. According to what is presented in most porn, there are two separate models for making sound during sex, one for women and one for men. Porn teaches us that women are supposed to have wild, screaming orgasms at the slightest touch. In contrast, the model for men is one of mostly silence, maybe letting out the occasional grunt or the cliché, "Oh yeah, baby."

Clearly, neither of these models is helpful. Sound doesn't need to be just about performance, nor does it have to be stifled and shut down. Rather, sound can be both an expression and an exploration of what you are feeling.

When I broke through in terms of making sound, it added a whole new dimension to the sexual experience. I had previously been in the "silent man" category, and I have questioned why that was. Was it because I learned as a teen to masturbate silently so my parents wouldn't hear me? Was it because I was ashamed of sex and pleasure such that I couldn't let myself express real enjoyment? Was it because as a boy I learned to not outwardly express emotion or feeling? Was it because I was generally disconnected from my body and living in my head, and thus not feeling anywhere near as much as she was? The truth is, all of these probably played a role in my silence.

I learned a lot about making sounds during sex from the women I was with. They would moan and scream and make all sorts of noises while I was just quiet. In retrospect, this wasn't very fair to them. Have you ever had a time when, let's say, you were going down on her, and she just laid there not making a sound while you were lapping away between her legs, giving it all you've got? How did that feel to you?

I have experienced this before, and I would question myself: *Is she enjoying this? Am I doing something wrong? Maybe I should do something different.* But no matter what I did to improve the situation for her or try to create more pleasure for her, she would just remain quiet. Contrast that experience to being with a woman who made enthusiastic sounds while you were going down on her. Which experience was more fun? Which encounter did you desire to do again? Which one was a really enjoyable experience for you?

When you make sounds that indicate to her that what she is doing is pleasurable for you, you provide moment-by-moment feedback to her that you are enjoying her. Sex becomes more fun and dynamic for both of you, and she wants to do it. Your sounds act as a form of reward to her, which inspires her to do it more. This is why I have come to cheekily refer to sound as the secret to getting more blow jobs!

When I first started getting the hint that there was something here for me to explore through sound, I was really insecure about the idea of making any noises during sex. I was afraid that I would look or sound silly or that it would be a turnoff for her. Maybe she would even laugh at me. So I started subtly, quietly, under my breath. Barely audible utterings and whispers: "Mmmmm . . ." Even with this minor approach, I noticed her positive reaction: a smile on her face as I found my way to making sound.

As my lover received positive feedback that I was enjoying her sexuality, I could see that it obviously felt good to her, too. She opened into the experience even more, and as she did, I let myself make a little bit more sound. It was slow going at first, and I was initially quite insecure about it, but the more I gave myself permission to get into the sounds, the more positive a response she had. Together, this created a highly rewarding—and hot!—feedback loop.

I slowly started actively exploring my vocabulary of sounds, different kinds of sounds, different kinds of moaning and tonality. Some of my favorites now are guttural growls and animalistic roars, as these sounds taught me how to more directly tap into primal, animalistic energies.

As she feels that animal aspect come out of me, it often gives her permission to unleash more of her inner animal, as well. Over time and through exploration,

I discovered all of these fun games we could play together with sound, games like animalistic call-and-response. She would make a sound with her exhale, and as she inhaled, I would make a sound in response, then she would make her next exhale with a sound. It was as if these growls and noises were the language of our primal bodies communicating with one another without saying a word.

Sound moves energy. Sound *is* energy. Music is sound waves moving through the air. I learned that I could use my sounds to further disperse the sexual energy or move it from one place to another in my body. For example, I could use sound to spread the energy in my groin throughout my whole body.

We can see our human instinctual drive to make sound in the example of a toddler running down the hallway screaming and wailing and making all sorts of sounds. Why? Because it feels good. He is releasing and moving energy with his entire body through sound.

In contrast to our instinctual drive to make sound, we can look to the cultivated ancient discipline of martial arts. When a martial artist makes a punch, it is always accompanied by a particular loud exclamation that is used to concentrate the energy of that movement. This is done with the knowledge that the sound intensifies the force and the precision of the movement. An intentional concentration of energy is forced out through the fist. A specific sound is made because it strengthens the velocity and impact of a particular punch. Martial artists channel energy out from the core through the fist because they are trained to know that sound can be an explosive and potent way of moving energy.

Perhaps this is obvious, but it is important to understand that breath and sound work hand in hand. Similar to the martial artist channeling energy from the core, you can use slow, deep inhalations to draw energy up and out from your pelvis, and then use sound to help it further shoot through your body. The key here is not to simply focus on what to do when you are about to come; that is plan B. Plan A is to keep the sexual energy circulating throughout your body at all times, and in doing so, notice your lover's response.

Allow your sounds to be an exploration of what you are feeling. You may think, *Well, I don't know what kind of sound to make.* Make any sound at all, and observe it as you are making it. How does it feel? Does it feel like it is adding a quality or dimension to your sexual experience? Does it feel right in your body? If not, try something else.

Play with pitches. Move from higher to lower pitches, and experiment with different tones. If you are familiar with the yogic tone of *OM*, try bringing this into your lovemaking. Experiment with mimicking different types of animal sounds. Different types and pitches of sound vibrate in different parts of your body, and you can create sounds from different parts of your body. You will notice how different it feels when you make sounds from your throat as opposed to when the sound comes from deep in your belly, or even from your balls.

I have come to think of the ability to express vocally as being a litmus test for our degree of freedom and liberation. How fully expressed are you? When you make sounds, sexually or otherwise, how restricted do you feel? Or how free? Do you find any discomfort in it? Can you just let yourself go? Are you worried that other people will hear you or what they will think? Are you able to connect to the more primal and animalistic sounds, and in so doing channel that energy and spirit from within you?

Do this on your own with your ESE practice so that you can let yourself get wild, or even silly, without worrying about what anybody else will think. Give yourself permission to play with this natural human expression and to find your pleasure in it—that is the key. The more you find your authentic pleasure in sound, the more at ease you will be with it and the easier it will be for you to take sound-making into your sex with other people.

With your sound, you can encourage her to build her own repertoire of sound, as well, which will add richness and depth to her experience. You will likely discover that the more you make sound, the more present and dropped into your body you will feel, the more control you will have over your sexual response, and the more pleasure you will both experience.

How easy or difficult is it for you to vocally express your pleasure? What kinds of sounds do you make during sex, if any? Add into your ESEs an intentional exploration of different kinds of sounds, from guttural growls to high-pitched tones and more. How does it affect what you are feeling?

38.
MOVEMENT: THE MOTION OF THE OCEAN

In high school, when my friend Yasmine heard that I couldn't dance, she responded, "That's ridiculous! Anyone can learn to dance." She told me to meet her at her locker at the end of the school day and she would teach me. Nervously optimistic, I dutifully showed up for my lesson. She put on her boom box and said simply, "Show me what you got." I just stood there awkwardly looking at her. After much prodding, I gave it a go. I was so completely caught up in my head and uncomfortable in my body that I don't think I hit a single beat. First she just looked at me, dumbstruck, then she burst out laughing. "I'm sorry, but I have no idea how to work with that." And so ended my dance lesson.

If I thought I was uncomfortable in my body and with the idea of dancing before, this experience made it ten times worse. Now I had external confirmation that I sucked, that I was a horrible dancer, and that there was nothing I could do about it, so I became exponentially more awkward.

I finally got over it after many years—with a little help from MDMA. I was introduced to psychedelic drugs (primarily ecstasy, mushrooms, and acid) when I was twenty-two years old and living in the Netherlands for six months. I stumbled into the Goa trance party scene. When I was on ecstasy (*molly* or *E*), all my inhibitions were gone. MDMA dropped me into my body and allowed me to move without thinking about how I looked to anyone else. In retrospect, I am sure that my movement was a bit clunky in the beginning, but I didn't care. I was high, having a great time, and finally feeling free in my body. I came to fall in love with dancing and letting the music move through me—eventually even when stone-cold sober.

What does this have to do with sexual self-mastery? Sexual self-mastery requires you to be both disciplined and free, to liberate your body from your mind, to let your body move, and to no longer be stiff in your movements but to let them be wildly expressed. In order to do that, you have to let go of any fears of how you look. You can refine it later, but first, get free. Express.

Easier said than done.

You may find it easy, or you may find it extraordinarily difficult. I have seen, time and time again at our Evolved Masculine retreats, that when we explore movement or dance, there are always some men who are incredibly stiff in their bodies and movements. They look around awkwardly to see what other guys are doing or to see if anybody is watching and judging them.

I have come to understand that a big part of the fear is in how we are perceived by others. Perhaps you don't like to dance because you feel like you don't do it well—and then you can't learn how to dance because you don't like it. This, of course, creates a self-defeating loop that you can't escape until you break free from identifying with how you look and focus on how you feel. (This is directly relatable to how you show up in sexual encounters, as well.)

Resistance can come from a fear of ridicule, of being perceived as gay or girly, or of being incompetent. Perhaps, like me, someone told you that you can't dance or that you are a shitty dancer, and you believed it as an immutable truth that became part of your identity.

For a lot of guys, dancing requires intoxication. They have a perceived need to release inhibitions in order to allow themselves to be free in their bodily expression. But whether we are speaking of alcohol or other drugs, this need can create either a master-slave relationship or a teacher-student relationship.

A master-slave relationship is one in which you come to believe that you need the intoxicating substance in order to dance, or have sex, or whatever it is you are using it for. The teacher-student relationship is one in which alcohol or some other substance helps you learn and open to a new way of being that you hadn't known before, one that you can become in touch with. You no longer need the teacher when you have integrated the change into your being.

I was asked many times during my Erotic Rockstar years how I kept my body in such great physical condition; I didn't go to the gym, and I didn't have a traditional exercise routine, yet I had rock-hard abs and was in phenomenal shape. My answer was always something along the lines of "a lot of dancing and a lot of sex, and approaching both of them as full-body activities."

With dance, especially in the festival environment, I learned to use my entire body. Sometimes both my hands and my feet were on the ground. I would engage my upper body by pushing off of a wall or hanging off a part of the stage structure or swinging on a pole—or, in one of my more epic Erotic Rockstar moments, acrobatically dancing upside down while dangling by the heel of one platform boot, twenty-five feet above a thousand people dancing in a geodesic dome at Burning Man.

Likewise, sex was more than simply going in and out, forward and back with my hips. It was crawling all over my lover, moving all across the bed, across the room, undulating my body, letting my arms, legs, and head thrash about as the waves of pleasure moved through me. There is a reason why sex is sometimes referred to as horizontal dancing.

Begin to explore letting your entire body move. This may come easy to you, or it might be incredibly challenging. Use your ESEs to actively push your edges of what is comfortable. Keep exploring until full-body movement becomes easier, and you will have an easier time bringing this level of movement into your sex with a partner.

One of the biggest mistakes that men make in sex is something called "piston fucking." Piston fucking is when men thrust their hips in and out along one axis. Your hips can move 360 degrees in all directions. When you learn to open up the range of motion within your hips and pelvis, a greater range of pleasure opens up for both of you. Additionally, having an expanded range of motion and movement helps your sexual energy move its way throughout your body.

As you begin to open your movement and subtly (or significantly) gyrate in different ways, you can visualize your cock inside of her. Visualize a map of the inside of her pussy. Use this tool to intentionally explore and stimulate different parts of the inside of her pussy with your cock, mapping each part. Know where you are in her pussy. Notice how she responds to different types of stimulation on different parts of her. Experiment with different levels of pressure and different speeds at different points in her arousal cycle. You will come to find commonalities across women and that there is much that makes each woman and her particular sexual response unique.

Allow the sensation that you feel in your groin to move through your limbs and your torso. Let your body move with the sensation, and feel the sensation rise along with that movement. Let your body move in whatever ways it wants to move.

Our modern, civilized society has socialized much of the animal out of most boys, from the age of five to eighteen. Sit in a chair, be still. Don't move for six hours a day, five days a week. Graduate. Sit at a desk in front of a computer. Sit behind the wheel of a car and drive. Sit on the couch and watch TV or play video games. This is not what we were made for. This society has massively depleted our wildness. Our passive lifestyle choices function brilliantly to diminish our instinctual and sexual nature. If you want to be an extraordinary lover, then you have to get in touch with and inhabit your body and its primal capacity for movement.

The Evolved Masculine path is about deepening empowerment and freedom. There is power and freedom in inhabiting your body and being free in your movement and expression. Freezing off and shutting down that place inside that lets desire move us is a learned cultural conditioning. Sexual self-mastery is an unlearning of that; we are relearning to be more human.

A lot of men are particularly tight in their hips, and that tightness restricts the natural flow of sexual energy. You are now training your body to shift from your pelvis being the container of your sexual energy to your entire body being the container. We need to open up your initial container and make it easier for that energy to flow. That means opening your hips and creating more mobility in your spine. Yoga can be incredibly helpful for this, as can anything that opens up your hips and spine. The more movement you have in your hips and spine, the easier your sexual energy can flow throughout your body. Swivels, or figure-eight motions with your hips, create ease and mobility in your spine and openness in your hips, which will help that energy move. Self-massaging your pelvis, hips, glutes, and hamstrings will also help a lot.

Tantric sexual teachings include what are known as *kriyas*. These little jolts of kundalini release are quick pulses of energy that move through your system.

They have their own mini-orgasm-type feel to them. To the uninitiated, a kriya can look a little like a spasm or sudden jolt of your body.

I think of kriyas as a collaborative experience. The energy wants to move, and you must say yes and allow it. There may be ways that you are unconsciously stopping this type of energetic release. Allow it to happen. Kriyas can happen most easily when you are in the early stages of this process, as they break through old energetic blocks. They can be subtle to notice at first, so I suggest allowing yourself to overdo your movements.

Put on some music that feels good to you. Close the door, and in the privacy of your own space, with nobody else around, practice letting your body move. It does not matter at all what you look like. This important first step is to learn to let yourself move without restriction, without fear, without holding yourself back in any way. Overdo your movements. Let your hands sway over your head. Shake out the stiffness in your body. Try doing your ESE standing, and let yourself move about the room.

Another way you can use movement to help your sexual energy flow is through undulating your spine like a snake. If you have ever seen a woman intensely arch her back while experiencing sexual pleasure, whether in person or on video, she is unconsciously helping the sexual energy move up her spine. You can create waves with your spine so you are not just arching but rather fully undulating, creating a rolling of the spine.

You can also use your hands and your physical touch to help move this energy out from your groin. While you are in an aroused state, grasp your hands around the base of your cock and physically pull down the insides of your thighs. Grab again around the base and pull up, spreading this energy throughout your torso.

On a physiological level, you are engaging your nervous system through these actions. With the buildup of sexual energy, the nerve endings in your genitals light up. Taking your attention and awareness up out of your cock and moving those sensations throughout your body will light up more and more of your nervous system in the process. For added fun, your lover can do this to you, as well, just as you can use your hands to help spread her sexual energy.

Do you steer clear of the dance floor? Have you gotten negative feedback about your moves? Try abandoning the old narrative about yourself and just move with the music, alone or with a partner. Try this exercise as a prelude to sex or ESE. In your ESEs and sexual experiences, practice allowing your entire body to move and explore.

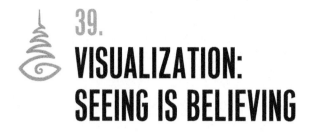

39.
VISUALIZATION: SEEING IS BELIEVING

I was in my junior year at New York University, spending the spring semester abroad in Madrid, Spain. My girlfriend, Mia, also in the program, was experienced with psychedelics, while I had never experimented with anything other than marijuana. I felt comfortable with her and decided that I was going to pop my psychedelic cherry, so to speak, for my twenty-first birthday.

We sat on a park bench on a gorgeous lake in Madrid, and we each ingested an eighth of an ounce of psilocybin mushrooms. About forty minutes later, I began to see halos forming on the lights around us and streaks of light shooting out in different directions from the headlights on the cars passing in the distance. I remember saying to Mia, "If this is all there is to it, I already think it is amazing." The experience punctured my notion of reality. I was seeing things I had never seen before in my twenty-one years of life. All my notions of reality came into question. *Are these halos and streaks of light always there, and I'm just not normally able to perceive them? What else is real that I have written off due to my own inability to perceive it?*

I was in utter awe as I lay back on the grass and stared up into the branches of the tree above us, then closed my eyes and witnessed a fractal-pattern laser-light show playing out across the movie screen of my mind.

I started to experience my body in a new way. I would have moments of feeling like my body was translucent and that there were fiber optic lights networked throughout my entire body. As I moved in different ways, different sections and pathways would light up accordingly. As I breathed in, they would glow brighter, and as I exhaled, they would dim. It was as though there was an energetic field around me and in me that had its own pulse, expanding and contracting, expanding and contracting.

Years later, I came across Alex Grey's iconic paintings, visual representations of the energetic body. Instantly I thought, *That! That's what I felt! That's what I was in touch with!*—the glow emanating out beyond the physical edge of the body, the blur between where I ended and the rest of existence began.

Seeing Grey's paintings and the way he detailed the energetic system made it easier for me to tap into the energetic system, to see it in my mind's eye, and to map my now-clearer visualization of it onto my own body—and with that, to be able to feel my energetic system more fully.

> You can see Alex Grey's painting *Psychic Energy System* at: http://www.alexgrey.com/art/paintings/sacred-mirrors/alex_grey_14_psychic_energy_system

Though my initial connection to the energetic body came through psychedelics and festival party environments, I sought out what the ancient mystics had been exploring and writing about since the beginning of recorded history. For thousands of years, mystics have spent time in deep study and committed practice, and while there is strong evidence that psychoactive plants have played a pivotal role in accessing these visionary states—as with my experience—mystics also found these connections without using any substances.

This realization inspired me to delve more intently into the power of visualization and how it could (and definitely did) deepen my relationship to my sexuality without having to rely on ed psychedelic states to do so. While psychedelics and MDMA certainly helped me to find a deep connection to my energetic body, to visualize it in my mind's eye and therefore to feel it, I no longer require these substances in order to connect. I have the map now.

Even as I write this, I stop and bring my attention inward. I can find the pulse of the energetic movement when I bring my two palms to face one another, about six inches apart. Just as the heartbeat has its pulse and the breath has its pulse, this movement of energy in my body has its own pulse, as well.

In middle school I was obsessed with playing *Street Fighter 2* at my local arcade. The main character, Ryu, had a special move where, if you swung the joystick down, down-forward, forward, and hit a punch button—*HA-DO-KEN!*—he would create a large ball of energy, forced out through his hands, and push it at his opponent, inflicting damage. We can see these mystical depictions of "balls of energy," or rays of streaming light, throughout popular culture. These symbolic representations, even when seen in cartoons or video games, have roots in something real. Eastern traditions have been studying and practicing the connection to the energetic body and energetic fields for millennia.

While sensing energy involves attuning yourself to subtlety, sexual energy is arguably the most tangible, the strongest, and the most powerful. Through the practice of visualizing energy building in your sex, and then using your intent and the will of your mind's eye, you can imagine moving that energy into different parts of your body—particularly in conjunction with the other tools of breath, sound, and movement. Imagining this energy moving while using your breath, sound, and the movements of your body makes feeling and moving the energy easier.

Let's demystify the word *visualization*. For the uninitiated, visualization can be difficult to wrap your head around. Simply put, visualization means to see in your mind's eye, to imagine. We actually do this all the time. Little children are fantastic at it. They play make-believe and games of imagination constantly. Somewhere along the way, though, most of us ended up learning that imagination is kids' stuff and that "it's time to get serious." But imagination is the tool we use to create new possibility in our lives.

At its most basic, visualization is a tool that will help you move energy, including sexual energy, throughout the body. The invitation is to practice visualizing this energy in whatever way works for you: a white light, a little ball of energy, or fiber optics that light up as they are touched. The important aspect is to be able to see it in your mind's eye. Over time, as you are able to hold in your mind's eye the visual qualities of the energy you experience in your body, feeling it will become easier.

The unconscious mind doesn't create a separation between what you see in the psyche and what is happening in external reality, or "real life." This means that you have the ability to literally build neural pathways through your body by imagining them. Visualize and build the capacity to see this sexual energy as it is being generated in your groin, then spreads from your pelvis and throughout the rest of your body. Use your mind's eye to observe it spreading from your pelvis up your torso to your shoulders. Now send the energy down your arms and out your fingertips. Finally, draw this energy from the torso up through the neck, out the top of the head, and through your eyes and mouth, nostrils and ears. Visualizing this energy will help the nerve endings throughout your body know that they are to fire along with the nerve endings in your groin.

As you play with visualization, practice taking slow, deep breaths. Instead of just focusing on the breath coming in through your nose or mouth and into your lungs, imagine that this energy is moving from your groin up your spine and out through the limbs of your body as you breathe. As you make sound, imagine seeing and feeling the energy disperse and move with the feeling of the sound's vibration in your body.

Initially, you may just be imagining the flow, but as you visualize it repeatedly over time, you will not only see this flow of energy in your mind's eye but also develop a felt sense of it. Remember, neurons that fire together wire together. Practice and play with it. Through repetition, connecting to the subtleties of your energetic body will become increasingly easier.

I know that when I started, I found playing with energetic visualizations quite difficult. I wasn't sure if I was doing it right. At most, I would see little flashes, which sometimes discouraged me, yet I found that through practice and repetition over days, weeks, months, and years, it became increasingly easy. I began to see these pathways of energy in my body more clearly, and to establish a deeper understanding of how to use my imagination to expand the energy throughout my body. Now I can't not see this energy moving through my body.

Visualization has profoundly changed how I make love. Whether I am with my wife or by myself, an intense flow of energy streams from my cock and balls throughout my body with each breath. With each exhalation, I can use the mapping of my energetic pathways to send energy out through my cock and to push energy into my lover's pussy and up through her body with every thrust. The more energetically sensitive and tuned in she is, the more she is able to feel this force of energy penetrating and radiating throughout her entire body. Even the less-attuned woman will usually feel something, even if she can't quite understand or explain what she is feeling.

Visualization and imagination are powerful tools of creation. As a core tool of energetic self-mastery, a visualization practice allows you to understand and connect to the multidimensional energetic pathways within your system. By mapping your own energetic fiber optics, you can connect in much deeper, more potent ways with your own sex, and therefore, with your lover.

Do you have a story that says you aren't very good at visualization? If so, are you willing to let that story go, be patient with yourself, and enjoy the process? The next time you have sex, either with yourself or with a partner, try visualizing the energy. Visualize the sexual energy in your groin, and imagine that your inhales build it. On your exhale, use the power of your imagination to spread the energy from your pelvis out through your limbs, torso, and head. Practice it repeatedly until you have the hang of it.

40.
BEYOND EJACULATORY CHOICE: THE FOUR GATES OF SEXUAL SELF-MASTERY

Once you have integrated the four tools and walked through the first gate of ejaculatory choice, the other three gates of sexual self-mastery will be much closer than you realize.

Full-Body Orgasms

Men tend to relate to orgasms as something that takes place in their dicks. Full-body orgasms make those types of orgasms feel like nothing more than a sneeze, a buildup of pressure in your pelvis, and then *achoo!*—out flies your snot. Full-body orgasms, on the other hand, are experienced throughout your entire body.

If you want to have full-body orgasms, you have to train your system that the entire body is part of your sexual experience. You can train your nervous system so that all of the nerve endings of your body light up with pleasure.

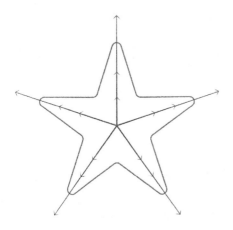
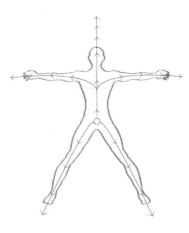

Think of your body like a starfish. Your sex is the center. Your legs and arms are the limbs of the starfish, and the rest of your torso and head is the fifth limb. Generate the sexual energy from your cock, and as it builds in the pelvis, use the four tools to spread the energy outward to the tips of your starfish, and even out through the tips. *Generate and spread. Generate and spread.* As you do this more and more, you will open up the energy channels of your body, and your orgasms will begin to explode out from your sexual center, down your legs and out the bottoms of your feet, up your torso, down your arms and out your fingertips, and up your neck and through the top of your head. This is a powerful, full-body orgasm.

Non-Ejaculatory Energetic Orgasms (NEO)

I was taught that orgasm and ejaculation were the same thing for men. When I first heard about non-ejaculatory orgasms, I found the idea hard to grasp, as do some of the men I work with. However, most of us have had the opposite experience at some point. You ejaculated, but it would be a stretch to call it an orgasm, as it wasn't particularly pleasurable. So there: you have experienced ejaculation and orgasm as two separate things. Now we just have to focus on doing it the other way around.

Let's define *ejaculation* as the expulsion of semen, the fluid itself, and *orgasm* as a flood of pleasure and energy moving through the body. NEOs are the experience of that flood of peak pleasure and energy through the body without the ejaculation.

I like ejaculatory orgasms. I like them a lot. They are one of life's great pleasures–and I still argue that there are benefits to viewing ejaculatory orgasms as just one of the options available to you in your sexual repertoire.

I know plenty of colleagues who are truly *anti*-ejaculation, so I want to make clear that I am very much *not* that. Besides liking the feeling personally, I consider my work to include alleviating sexual shame, guilt, and fear. Penalizing men for ejaculating simply gives us a different thing to feel guilt or shame about.

One reason to develop the ability to orgasm without ejaculating is to expand your sexual palette, the flavors and experiences that are available to you when you go into any sexual experience. Ejaculatory orgasm is one expression available to you, but not the only one.

Another good reason to develop this skill is to prevent the drop in energy that most men experience after they ejaculate. Also, as men get older, the energetic loss that comes with ejaculation tends to get more pronounced, and it takes longer to get hard again. (The time between erections, called the *refractory period*, typically becomes extended throughout a man's life.)

A lot of athletes, especially pro athletes, don't have sex the night before a game because they believe it affects their performance. I propose that if you were having NEOs instead, then your performance would likely improve. Non-ejaculatory, energetic orgasms don't make you want to roll over and fall asleep like ejaculatory orgasms do. Instead of feeling drained from your energy exploding out of you, you can keep going as a result of the implosion in you, which draws the sexual energy up through your whole body. You may even be harder than you were before. So, reader, if you are an athlete, test this out, and if you hit more home runs, goals, or touchdowns, send me a message.

Personally, I have found that my sweet spot is running my sexual energy every day but ejaculating about once a week. I find that my energy throughout the week tends to be the best with that rhythm. When I have a NEO or engage in non-ejaculatory sex, I carry that energy with me throughout the day. I feel more lit up, alert, and alive. I feel that animalistic drive in me much more, especially now that I can enjoy it without feeling overwhelmed by it and feeling like I need to do something to get rid of it.

The simplest way to describe how to have a NEO is to use your now-strengthened PC muscles to create a seal that prevents the ejaculation while simultaneously using the four tools to channel the intensity of sensations up through your body. The key is in getting the timing right. Based on my experience teaching these skills for more than a decade, I will add that the timing is likely earlier than you think it is. Keep testing it until you get the delectable reward.

Male Multiple Orgasms

Once you are experiencing non-ejaculatory orgasms, having multiple orgasms should come easily (pun intended). With the implosion of energy up through your body, you will likely feel more energized than you were before the orgasm, and with that, you can keep on going, riding wave after wave of orgasmic pleasures along with your lover.

Men can have many different kinds of multiple orgasms, just as women can. You can have one NEO, continue having sex, and then have an ejaculatory orgasm. You can have one orgasm that rolls into another that rolls into another. You can have a NEO that then dips your sexual energy a bit, then build that sexual energy back up and have another, and cycle through that a few times. You can have a few NEOs and then end your raucous romp with an ejaculatory orgasm. Or you can simply have a few NEOs and come to a point of feeling done and fully satiated without ever ejaculating.

As you travel further along your path of sexual self-mastery, the available options of sexual expression continue to expand. This deepening of your connection with your own body will provide you with far greater pleasure, make you a more extraordinary lover, and transform your ability to both understand and feel into the women in your life.

Have you crossed the threshold to any of the four gates of sexual self-mastery? Do you believe it is possible? Do you believe it is possible for YOU? The path of sexual self-mastery is a commitment. It takes time and dedication, and the results are worth it. Make the commitment, have patience with yourself, and walk the path.

PART 4

UNDERSTANDING WOMEN AND THE FEMININE

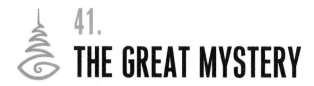

41.
THE GREAT MYSTERY

Meeting Kirsten was like encountering an entirely new type of creature. Her life was about beauty, creative expression, dance, flow, and letting the wind take her into the magic and mystery of life. She was open to receiving what the world has to offer, and she felt *everything* so, so much. To this day, she is one of the most embodied beings I have ever met.

Kirsten worked with her body all day and night, and her idea of fun in her downtime was stretching and craft projects. Much of her life was made up of trapeze, stilt walking, contact juggling, dancing, and playing dress-up. She would adorn herself in wild circus makeup and skimpy, shimmery outfits, and revel in her sensual expression. I was in awe of her and completely fascinated by her world. The way in which she experienced life was so unlike my own.

We had incredible passion in our relationship. We had intense, exhibitionistic sex in front of hundreds of people. We would make love on set for professional erotic photographers and camera crews just for fun. We made live erotic performance art together.

And she drove me mad.

I didn't understand why she did the things she did. Some of the choices she made ran counter to anything I would imagine as logical. I just wanted to understand her. *Why is she like that? What the hell does she want from me? Why does she seem so crazy sometimes?* Her emotions were all over the place; she could go from being intensely sexy one moment to being deeply angry the next, to laughing out loud, to crying in tears . . . and if I played my cards right, to ecstatic orgasm—all in the span of an hour or less. Often.

I didn't understand why we fought so much. *What does she want from me?* She seemed to need something that I didn't know how to provide. I loved her so much, and I just wanted her to be happy. I wanted things to be easier. I wanted *her* to be easier, but something always upset her, no matter what I did. While I could sometimes get her back to a place of happiness, she would explode in a grenade of tears and fairy sparkle again a day or two later. I didn't understand; I would have done anything to understand. My love for her was so deep that when things weren't working, I felt a deep anguish—I could not get this right, and I so, so wanted to get it right.

This unpredictability launched me into a deep exploration of the dynamics at play in our relationship, not simply as the personal identities of "Destin" and "Kirsten," but more so as a "man" and a "woman." Even in my heightened state of fucked-up-ness, I strapped on my inner professor goggles and entered intense research-and-development mode, delving into different lenses about relationships and discovering something called *polarity*. Polarity is a way of looking at relationship based on the idea that the masculine and the feminine are two different energetic poles. Like magnets, they both attract and repel.

I rapidly and repeatedly tested in my relationship with Kirsten all that I was learning from different relationship teachings and styles. I explored extensively, both that which resonated and that with which I vehemently disagreed.

Part of the intense exploration of my masculinity was rooted in my desire to better understand Kirsten and the new-to-me meta concept of *the feminine. If I want to understand women, I need to understand what the feminine is. What is at the root of the differences between us?* Kirsten certainly seemed to be connected to something that I simply had no direct access to. I didn't understand, but I was fascinated. I was determined to understand this otherworldly way of living and being.

The deeper I went into my exploration and understanding of the masculine, the better I began to understand the feminine through the contrast itself. Similarly, the more I explored the feminine, the deeper I understood the masculine. I arrived at a point where I started to see these masculine and feminine energies stream and express through people—including myself—regardless of gender, similar to the ways in which Neo in *The Matrix* came to see multidimensional streams of code.

I wanted to understand my masculine, but I didn't want to do so at the expense of the qualities I associated with my feminine, which I had come to appreciate as an essential part of me. I found that if I brought conscious awareness to this self-discovery process, I could explore all of it. I had wounds around my masculine aspect, yet I also held wounds around my feminine.

Ever since I was a boy, I heard messages such as, "Don't throw like a girl" and "What are you? A pussy? Fucking faggot!" All of those messages told me to suppress, dominate, or kill off the feminine that existed within me. Since then, I have come to want to understand *her*, the feminine within me, and how to draw from that energy as I choose to, not retreat into it because of fear of my masculine or wounds that I still hold.

The more I came to understand and appreciate the feminine *within* myself, the easier it was for me to understand and appreciate the feminine *outside* of myself—the feminine in her, in the women around me, even the feminine in other men. So long as I judged the feminine within me, some part of me, however unconscious, was judging the feminine in women.

I was learning, but not quickly enough to save my relationship with Kirsten. I must have made an internal decision to deeply understand women and the feminine because I didn't ever want to experience such pain again. I didn't ever want to be hurt like that again. I didn't ever want to lose the woman I loved again.

While my path was long and winding, I was in fact coming to understand a lot about women and the feminine, and not just intellectually. Rather, I was integrating my lessons into my body through lived experience. When I would read or hear something, I would check to see how it felt in my body and whether it was resonant with my value system. If it passed that inquiry, I would then test it in my interactions with women. I realized that I was on to something, not simply by the number of women who eagerly came to share my bed, but more so by the way they spoke about their experiences and time with me, and by and large, how they continue to relate to me to this day.

This is not to say that I have it all figured out. I don't. Honestly, I don't expect to *ever* have women 100 percent figured out, nor do I want to. Part of my masculine nature is driven to understand and solve. *Would she be so fascinating if you had her completely figured out?*

The more deeply sourced in her feminine she is, the more completely different way of experiencing the world she has. My hope is that you will come to a greater understanding of the women in your life and to orient yourself toward a deeper exploration of the feminine, to seek to better understand it in all women—and not just to figure out how to get what you want.

Certain indigenous tribes refer to their notion of God as "The Great Mystery." I love this phrase; as long as humanity has been around, we have sought to understand this existence. *Life. Who are we? Why are we here? What is all this?* We have spent all of humanity trying to understand, and we understand only a fraction of what there is to know; yet look at how far we have come! Assuming we survive, a thousand years from now what we know will be far beyond anything we can comprehend today, and still it will be a tiny fraction. However, it is clearly a worthy, if endless, pursuit.

This is how I relate to the feminine. She will always be a mystery. There will always be that which we can't understand, yet spending one's life seeking to understand her more is a worthy and fulfilling goal.

In the early 2000s, *STA Travel* had banner ads on the sides of buses in San Francisco that read, "Do something great for your country. Leave." As someone who had already done significant travel, I loved this ad, though I questioned how much it was understood by those who hadn't yet traveled. Leaving the United States and experiencing other cultures led me to see and understand my own country and culture in a new and deeper way. I was positively influenced by my contact with other cultures and completely different ways of seeing the world and living life—and I brought these new understandings back with me to my home country.

Likewise, leaving the native land of your masculine nature as you journey into the mysterious realm of the feminine will only help you more deeply understand yourself and your own masculinity, and it will make your experience of life itself that much richer. If your process is anything like mine, you will not only understand women more, you will have greater fulfillment in your relationship to women, and you will experience a fundamentally ing and evolutionary effect, as well.

What messages have you received about the feminine? How do you feel about the more feminine parts of yourself? How well do you think you understand women and the feminine? What aspect of Her do you find most baffling and wish you could better understand?

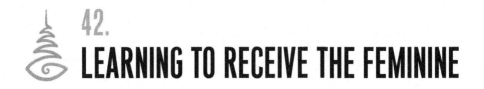

42.
LEARNING TO RECEIVE THE FEMININE

There is a creation mythology within tantric philosophy that I have been particularly influenced by and enamored with. In this story, Shiva, the masculine element of the Divine, represented as consciousness itself, and Shakti, the feminine element, represented as pure energy, come into sacred union, make love, and birth all of existence. I find the non-hierarchical, equitable notions of masculine and feminine in this context to be in stark contrast to the patriarchal male God-in-the-sky of the Judeo-Christian culture that I grew up in. Consciousness is neither better than nor more important than energy. Energy is not superior to consciousness. They are two halves of a whole, and together life and existence came to be.

The first time I encountered an explanation of masculine and feminine was within the context of a college sociology class that informed us that there had long been an argument about nature versus nurture. Either masculinity and femininity are innately determined by our biology or they are simply concepts constructed by our societies.

My lens is neither biological nor sociological, but rather, an energetic one. Masculine and feminine are energies that permeate the universe. All of it is accessible to anyone. There can be no masculine without the feminine and no feminine without the masculine, just as there can be no light without dark, no up without down, no positive magnetic pole without the negative magnetic pole.

The perspective I hold is that each of us does have an underlying core essence and that the vast majority of the time that core essence aligns with one's biological sex. However, this does not mean that your gendered identity is all that you are and all that you are supposed to express. There is an infinite array and combination of gendered potentiality that could express through each of us, man or woman.

As a culture, we don't understand the feminine, and history has shown us all too clearly that that which we do not understand we often oppress. What I have experienced through my own encounter of the feminine has blown my mind and changed me at a foundational level. When I first came into direct experience with the unashamed, fully expressed, full ownership of the feminine in all its magic, wildness, and beauty, my concepts of reality were blown apart.

Women who are deeply sourced in their feminine experience the world different from the way men (and women) who operate from their masculine do. The reason why some men think *she's crazy* is because they are expecting her to experience the world the same way they do, which makes sense given that the structures of this industrialized world were built from a masculine perspective. She has learned how to operate within this masculine-structured world and has adapted to it to an incredible degree, but one of the reasons why she may be perceived as "crazy" is because she is living in a world that was not made for her.

This completely different way of experiencing the world through the feminine contains a gift for us as men. It can add much richness to your life. Conversely, however, I believe that our lack of understanding and appreciation of the feminine is driving us toward destruction—again, not because masculinity and masculine perspectives are inherently destructive. When something is out of balance because you prioritize one set of values and principles while relegating the other as inferior, it will, by extension, organically create distortion in both. There simply has been no balance between the masculine and feminine, and this long-running imbalance is destructive, just as being out of balance in your personal life for a long time is a slow-moving train wreck: it can function for a while, but over time, shit starts to fall apart. But this is the water we swim in, similar to how, until you leave America, you can't really understand America.

Contrary to some opinions, I believe we are still at the very beginning of an upheaval that will be so fucking total that we will not be able to recognize the world anymore. This realignment of masculine and feminine on the planet is not simply about getting more women into CEO positions or electing a female President of the United States (though I welcome both); it is about a complete restructuring of our societies so they have roots that place feminine value systems, perspectives, and needs truly on par with their masculine counterparts. I have no idea how long it will take, and I have only little glimpses as to what that will look like, yet all I have seen and experienced has led me to stand firmly in the belief that this rebalancing is the foundational solution to much of what ails our planet.

A measure of one's masculinity is his ability to receive the feminine.

— **Rion Kati,** *Archetypal Allure Consultant*

During my relationship with Kirsten, I remember us leaving my apartment in Oakland and heading to the BART station. I was in a rush. (I am not sure if there was a reason for me to be in a rush or if it was simply habit.) I grabbed her hand and tried to move as quickly as we could to get there. She stopped suddenly, almost jerking my shoulder out of the socket in the process, and with a big smile on her face, showed me some beautiful flowers on the side of the road. She encouraged me to lean in and inhale their scent. At first I felt irritated. *We're on a mission. We're getting to the BART station. We've got somewhere to go!* But as I breathed in that lush and intoxicating fragrance, I quickly melted. *Wow.* I don't know how many times I had passed through that same way to go to the train, but I had never noticed those flowers before and wouldn't have even known they were there.

This would prove to be one of countless times Kirsten shared the beauty of this world with me: pointing out a mural on the side of the building, stopping whenever we were going somewhere so we could spend fifteen minutes watching the sun drop below the horizon, bringing my attention to the ways in which she would match her socks to her earrings to create an aesthetic balance to a look she had clearly put much thought into. Creating beauty and noticing the beauty in the world is a natural expression of the feminine, and one that was notably missing from my overly intellectualized, analytical, results-focused way of being.

Noticing beauty is part of my life now. I also know quite clearly that I am so aware of and appreciative of the beauty in this world because Kirsten and many women since were naturally much more aware of it and made a point to share it with me.

Thankfully, I allowed myself to open and be receptive to her sharing. I could have pushed it away. In that moment with the flowers, I could have snapped, "Not now. We're late!" But thankfully, I let it in, and my life is so much richer and more fulfilled as a result.

As men, we are learning how to receive the feminine and the gifts women have to bring into our lives beyond the sexual. A lot of men have a hard time with this, as it can bring up fear of engulfment: a loss of self or a loss of power—or both.

I have to be the one leading and making it happen. My job is to penetrate and have impact on her. If it needs to be that way all the time, where is the opening in us as men? Where is the opportunity for men to experience and receive the gifts that women have to bring to the conversation, to our sex lives, to our beings and growth processes?

My wife, Elie, has brought so much into my life in part because I have been in the practice of receiving it. She has taught me the value of slowing down. I have spent my life going from 0 to 100 in 2.2 seconds, racing through life, and I learned the hard way, through health crisis, that I can't sprint through life forever. She has taught me to balance my yang with yin, to let go, slow things down, and just be.

Nature does not hurry, and yet everything is accomplished.

— Lao Tzu

The women in my life have taught me so much. Loving women through the different chapters of my lived experience has deepened my understanding and capacity to truly cherish the gifts and the storms of the feminine. It is through loving women that I have learned to get out of my head and instead listen to the intuitive wisdom of my body and connect to my heart. Women have shown me how to let myself feel all my feelings more fully and to express both my pleasure and my pain. It is through women (and especially through my marriage with Elie) that I learned about love, nurturing, children, family, and being authentically connected to and protective of nature and the Earth.

The more I opened up to listen to, understand, and receive what the feminine has to offer, the more enriched my life has become. As fulfilling as it is, it wasn't just her sexuality that had value to me. I learned to recognize, value, and take in *all* the gifts that the feminine has to bring into my life.

Who are the prominent feminine individuals in your life? Think about the last time you brushed off an expression of her feminine energy, as I normally did before the BART/flower experience. Next time, try consciously enjoying and nurturing that element in women, and you will begin to experience and appreciate the feminine energy. Welcoming the feminine energy will attract more of it into your life.

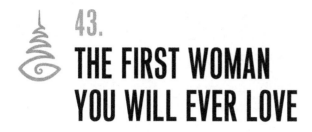

43.
THE FIRST WOMAN YOU WILL EVER LOVE

Like it or not, every single relationship you have in your life is impacted by the relationship you have with your mother.

I am writing this on the fifth anniversary of my mother's death. My mother was a morbidly obese woman, five foot four, 270 pounds. I spent most of my life embarrassed of her. Early on I picked up the message that having a fat woman as a mother was something to be ashamed of. Other kids would make fun of me about it, or they would make fun of her to my face. At the time, I did not have the confidence to stand up for her or myself.

My dad would call her a slob in front of my sister and me. By early childhood I had learned that my mom wasn't "the sharpest tool in the shed." By the time I was in fifth grade, I knew I was smarter than she was, which was of course reinforced by the many comments from my dad about my mother's low intelligence.

My mom couldn't hold a job, and most of the time she wasn't even looking. When she did get a (minimum wage) job, it would never last long. She would either quit or get fired within a few months. She would show up late one too many times or complain that standing on her feet hurt too much, and quit. For many years, I believed there was something wrong with my mother, that she had issues, and that, simply put, it was her fault she was the way she was.

In early adulthood, I learned that my mother carried more trauma than I had ever dared to imagine. When she was just five years old, she had contracted nearly fatal meningitis, which affected her cognitive development as well as her hearing (another thing that my dad, and eventually my sister and I, cruelly made fun of her for). She was the only child of my grandmother, who herself carried a lifetime of trauma as an Austrian Jewish Holocaust survivor. Additionally, my mom became pregnant when she was only a teenager and gave up her baby for adoption when she was just fifteen years old. This was in the early 1960s. I can only imagine the helplessness, fear, and grief this must have caused this young teenage girl, who would one day become my mother.

This knowledge catalyzed a shift in my awareness, from *There is something wrong with my mother* to *Holy fuck, no wonder life was so challenging for my mom—look at everything this woman has been through and survived.* Who wouldn't be traumatized from having endured these devastating experiences?

At thirty-four years old, while attending a weekend seminar (The Landmark Forum), I called my mother in accordance with an assignment we were given. I shared with her that as far back as I could remember, everybody in her life, including me, had been telling her she needed to lose weight. *You have to lose weight, you need to do it for your health. You have to do it for your family. Mom, you need to go on a diet.* This was a running refrain my mother was bombarded with, so many times, in so many different ways, yet over the last thirty years, I had known her to carry roughly the same amount of weight. At times she would lose as much as thirty pounds, but it wouldn't be long before it would come back, and then sometime later, the cycle would start again . . . and again . . . and again.

I realized during that powerful conversation that I wasn't willing to have a dysfunctional relationship with my mother anymore. I wasn't going to add to that constant voice in her head any longer. I told her that from that point onward, she would not hear those words come out of my mouth ever again. I committed to never asking her about her diet or speaking to her about her weight again. I no longer cared about her dieting or how many pounds she weighed. I accepted the fact that it was likely never going to change. My sole focus was on being a voice of unconditional love and unconditional acceptance of her exactly as she was. Nothing needed to change, ever. I was able to love and accept her as she was.

By setting my mother free and cutting the emotional umbilical cord to my need for her to lose weight in order for me to feel safe and loved, I set *myself* free. Radical acceptance of another may look like it is for them, but in truth, it is for *you.*

As I spoke those words, they were so utterly foreign to her that it was as though her psyche did not know how to compute this type of loving message. My mother was in her early sixties and had *never had anything like this said to her before.* I don't think she knew what to make of it. so she replied, "Look son, I know I need to lose this weight . . ." but I had to interrupt her. "Mom, I don't think you're getting what I'm saying. Your weight doesn't matter to me anymore, *you* do. You can carry this weight for the rest of your life, and I love and accept you exactly as you are. My love and acceptance of you has nothing to do with your weight, more, less, or staying the same. I accept you as you are."

A few months later, my mom was diagnosed with a rare form of leukemia, and a year later, she was dead. When we had that phone conversation, I had no way of knowing how little time I had left with her or that I would see her in person only one more time. I feel so fortunate that I was able to make peace with my mother in that last year, before she was gone forever. I know that so many sons and daughters never do.

There were so many things that bothered me about my mother for so long. Ultimately, I chose to not be another voice of conditional love in her world, another voice that constantly told her that in order to be accepted, she had to do or be something different. I have come to realize that this is the same pernicious message that many women struggle with: they must do or be something other than what or who they are in order to receive the love and acceptance they desire.

I have come to believe that most people who put on a lot of weight do so as a form of protection and that they are unconsciously using the weight to cover up their deep emotional scars. The weight isn't the primary issue, it is a symptom. My mother spent her life being criticized for the symptoms of her trauma instead of receiving support to move through the trauma itself.

The more I have come to understand trauma and its long-term effects, the more I have been able to find forgiveness and to cease blaming my mother for her imperfections and the mistakes that she made. I was given the opportunity to make peace with the realization that she was just doing the best that she knew how to, with what she knew at the time as a wounded young woman trying to figure out life for herself.

It has taken work, but I have come to a place of deep understanding and appreciation for all that my mother was for me throughout my life—especially for the profound, cosmic act of giving me life. Only now that I have been there, through my wife's pregnancy, witnessing her in labor and the serious miracle and intensity of giving birth, and seeing the breastfeeding and the day-in-day-out relentless sacrifice of being a mother, can I truly begin to fathom all that my mom did for me.

Because of the heartache my mother's weight caused her and all of our family, I have lived a life in which I continuously commit myself to rewiring my unhealthy patterns and directly confronting my deepest wounds. I have spent much of my adult life intentionally doing deep work on myself, attending workshops and seminars, and working with the best transformational coaches. Most people in the world do not have the drive toward self-mastery that I do. I now know that this is the gold of being the son of my mother, exactly as she was. I don't think it was a coincidence that I wasn't able to sustain a healthy, stable, loving relationship until I created a clearing for a new possibility of relationship with my mom.

Like it or not, unresolved issues with our parents are taken into all of our adult romantic relationships, and the imprint of our mother within our masculine system creates the mapping of how we create relationship in our lived experience. Until you deal with this with eyes open, it is going to continue to disempower you and wreak havoc on your life.

Until you make the unconscious conscious, it will direct your life and you will call it fate.

— Carl Jung

There are multi-faceted ways in which I expressed my mom's impact through my relationships with women. The most overt way was through what I have come to understand as the *rescuer-savior complex*. Because I spent the majority of my childhood unsuccessfully trying to "save" my mother from her complex trauma, I then carried this unconscious drive into my adult relationships with women. This looked like picking highly wounded women in the need of "saving" so that I had a function that could prove to me that I had worth and that I mattered.

The cost of this need was that my relationships were highly volatile and filled with drama and constant crisis, so that I was always in a position where I had to prove myself as worthy, although I was not conscious of this until many years later. Sex became a way that I could prove I was worthy to be accepted and loved. It required, however, that I constantly perform sexually, and I felt compelled to be an amazing lover not just for my own pleasure, but to earn my right to be loved.

The underbelly in all of this was a feeling of martyrdom; I felt like I had to constantly sacrifice my own needs for my lovers' and partners' needs and desires so that I could earn my position as needed and loved inside of the relationship. This painful dynamic ran rampant in my life until I understood its cause and was able to do work around my relationship with my mom, culminating in the day I called her to express my full acceptance of who she was, exactly as she was.

I have wondered if the work I do in the world does not have its root in Anjali's rape, after all, but perhaps started even younger, with my childhood desire to protect and save my mother and never having been able to.

Look, I know this isn't sexy, but my hope in sharing this vulnerable material with you is that you begin to understand the very real impact of the relationship you have with your mother, and the ways it will continue to cause chaos in your life until you can come to a place of peace and acceptance about who your mother truly is. This does not mean that you have to like her, or that you have to be in close relationship with her, but it does mean that coming into a place of acceptance of your mother as a *woman*, one who carries her own lived experience, wounding, trauma, and dashed hopes and dreams, will serve you on your path. What becomes possible from this place is an acceptance and a cherishing of *all* women for the truth of who they are, flaws, imperfections, and all.

What is your relationship to your mother like? Where are you withholding forgiveness for her? What do you imagine healing your relationship to your mother would open up for you? What would it take for you to truly forgive and come to a place of deeper understanding and appreciation of her?

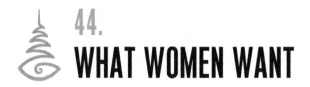

44.
WHAT WOMEN WANT

What *do* women want?

I have asked this question of a thousand women across multiple continents. I have crowd-sourced it on social media and asked it of women lying in my arms, naked bodies still glistening with sweat.

Like so many men, I have obsessed over this question throughout most of my life. So much of what I have come to understand came only through first getting it painfully wrong, hurting so much that I was committed to doing anything necessary to understand. Still today, there is more I don't understand than I do.

This question has quite literally been at the center of the insatiable quest of my personal and professional path. It has led me into the darkest of nights and my most testosterone-driven epic highs. And in pursuit of its answer, it has cost me thousands upon thousands of dollars, bringing me to the brink of bankruptcy *and* becoming the central axis of my life's work, earning me exponentially more than I ever had before.

To be able to get to what a woman wants requires patience and perhaps a bit of an archeological excavation. Women have been conditioned to tell you what she thinks you want to hear. She has likely been generationally entrained to share with you that which she thinks is acceptable for her to say or what seems possible to have. A woman who is courageous enough to share her desire with you will likely be in direct confrontation with not wanting to appear to be asking for too much or judged that she herself *is* too much.

At the same time, many men have a tendency to resist taking in the deeper truth of what women *do* communicate to them. As a result, women continue to feel frustrated and that they are not understood, sometimes believing that men don't care enough to *want* to understand.

Your Evolved Masculine mission, should you choose to accept it, is to gently but boldly strip away statements that come from fear, reflexive obedience to being "appropriate," or a cellular memory of *desire = danger*. The opportunity you have is to uncover her true desire, which runs underneath all of the cultural conditioning.

There is a way that you can continue to unconsciously crash around with this question, possibly judging and shaming women for being so complicated (or yourself for still not understanding). There is a way, however, that—perhaps for the first time—you can let this question truly enter your being.

What do women really want? That is the billion-dollar question, isn't it? What *do* women want?

Women want to be given the gift of themselves.

You are the key to unlocking the fullest, freest version of her that she can be. Women want you to know that—that you are the key to her deepest self—so you can *be* that, just as she is the key to your greatest version of self.

Giving a woman the gift of her self is in fact a form of devotion to her. The gift lies in your ability to call her into a greater, more expansive version of herself—without your ego, judgment, or expectation of what this may look like. Most women experience such an extreme deficit of feeling fully cherished for who and what they are that when you can create a container that uplifts a woman and helps set her free, you are in a powerful expression of leadership and service to her. You have the opportunity to create and be this for her, but only by first stepping beyond what you thought was possible for yourself and your life.

Tragically, far too many women go to their graves without ever having the experience of being wholly seen and adored. Not only have most of us not been taught how to open a woman in this way, but much of our cultural programming actually drives us in the opposite direction. *It doesn't have to be this way.*

Given the pervasive generational diminishment of women and the feminine in our history, women are still in the throes of learning how to be in relationship to their rapidly evolving sense of power. Here is the thing: opening a woman in this way is a learned skill. Yes, it requires you to build and sustain an evolved consciousness and capacity to hold high amounts of energy in your system, but that is why you are reading this book.

You can show her the possibility that exists within her, which she may not even know is there. You can draw it out from her, and she will rise and blossom into a fuller expression of herself. Women want—and crave—a man who is willing to invest in himself on all levels so that his very presence and beingness invites her to unfold into her most alive expression.

Women are mutable, paradoxical creatures; as the sky changes with a thousand shades of light, so does the nature of a woman. You can learn to meet her in every one of these expressions. If there is a foundational skill required to meet her in this way, it is your ability to see, hear, and feel her for who she is, as she is, moment to moment.

There are things that a woman wants, and there are things that a woman wants *from you*. She wants to be heard and listened to. She wants to know that her voice matters and that her thoughts, words, and opinions are valued. She wants to feel permission to be in her full expression, including her full sexual expression, without fear of being judged or fear for her physical and emotional safety.

She wants to be able to feel the full range of her feelings and emotions without being made wrong or needing to shut them down prematurely, or having a situation turn into her caretaking your emotional response to her feelings.

She wants to feel beautiful and know that you find her beautiful, that it is her, her essence underneath and beyond the skin, that is loveable and who you love. She needs to know that she can be an imperfect human being and that you can love the whole of who she is, inclusive of her flaws.

She wants to know that you care about what her most deeply held hopes and dreams are and that you will show up in full support of her reaching them. She desires to feel safe and free to explore herself and the world around her, and to know the parts of herself that she has yet to experience.

She longs to be held in her weakness as well as celebrated in her strength. She wishes to be fully at choice over her own body and what she does with it, including when and if to experience motherhood and what it is like to have a family.

She wants to be taken care of, yet not feel dependent on you. She desires to give to, nourish, and take care of you, yet not feel like she needs to be your mother. She needs to feel like you are in true partnership together, to be seen as a true equal—not the same as you but complementary and of equal value to you.

She wants her own actualization, to blossom into the fullness of who she is capable of becoming. She desires you in your full expression and actualization, and whatever your deepest truth is, to be it fully without holding back or apology. The more she experiences you as such, the more permission she feels to do and be the same.

She wants to experience being taken and led places that she can't get to on her own. She hungers to feel her desire for you and to feel your desire for her (and her specifically). She yearns to feel like she matters to you more than sex does, and she wants to be able to have the space to explore and discover her sexuality and her authentic sexual expression.

She desires a man who owns his masculinity and can penetrate her with his very being, with his energy and his gaze, long before the clothes ever come off. She craves being seduced, to be swept off her feet, to be whisked out from the mundane world of her day-to-day existence in all of its banality and experience adventure and wildness.

She wants to know that you are in command of your sexual energy, that you can unleash the animal within to ravish her, and that you can restrain that primal instinct in a moment—to both hold and release at will.

She wishes you to know her body even better than she does so she doesn't have to tell you what to do or what not to do, and yet to know that she could and that you would receive it easily and adjust accordingly without defense.

She craves to be free of her own shame, guilt, and fear; the more you can be free of yours, the more you give her permission to let it go, as well. She wants to discover the realms of her own sexual, pleasurable possibilities. She wants a man with whom she can explore and discover all of this.

Women's sexuality has been controlled for so long that she may not yet have had the opportunity to discover her sex in its authentic fullness. In very real ways, the Western woman is deep in the discovery of her authentic sexuality, sensuality, and expression. Who is she when she is not concerned about the church, what other people think, or how you judge her? Who would she be if she didn't have an internalized slut-shaming voice inside her head? Who would she be if she could follow her natural desire fully and without fear of retribution?

This is part of the immense value you are able to provide for a woman: to create a container of safety in which she can freely explore her own eroticism free of coercion or judgment, and to expand that container such that she continues to feel that safety and freedom in all aspects of her life.

Each of the above truths I learned through a combination of deep listening and trial and error. Even still, I am imperfect in meeting her in each of these desires. When I f, my life and my relationships simply do not work as well, thereby reinforcing the truth of these statements.

This is not about denying yourself and your own needs and desires. She wants you to know yourself ever more fully, to be able to stand in your own truth, to communicate, to hold your boundaries, *and* to strive to meet her desires.

I understand that reading all of this can feel overwhelming and intimidating. I share all of this with you not to place the responsibility of calling women into their fullness entirely on your shoulders. She certainly has her own responsibilities when it comes to her personal journey—and she can play a potent role in your activation, too. That said, if you desire to experience a woman in her most exalted expression, then the days of shirking your personal power and responsibility are over. Staying small and pretending that you are not a powerful being and an agent of evolutionary consciousness on this planet is believing a lie for the sake of comfort and your own distorted beliefs.

I do not share this information with you with the intention to present impossible standards that you can never attain and that would thereby reinforce all that is wrong with you, why you are undeserving, and why you will never be man enough to receive the love, sex, and attention you desire. This is not a list of everything you are supposed to already be. It is, however, an opportunity to see what is possible for you to grow into, day by day, year by year.

As you grow your capability in any one of these areas, your relationships will improve and she will open more fully in your presence. As you embrace her in her rise, your identity and context will shift because you will be called into the highest expression of your masculine aspect. She wants you to embrace her as she rises, because who you will become as a result of that process is everything she wants.

What one statement of what a woman wants most stuck out for you? What do you imagine would happen if you brought your attention to being a man who could help her have that single desire met? As you develop the experience and confidence in your ability to do so, bring your attention to the next of these desires. Take note of what changes in you in the process.

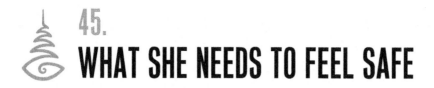

45.
WHAT SHE NEEDS TO FEEL SAFE

The average woman is smaller in both height and weight than the average man. Even if on one level she knows that you would never harm her let alone rape or murder her, there is another part of her that knows that if you wanted to, you could, and there would be nothing she could do to stop you.

Nothing.

Let that sink in for a moment.

If she has trauma in her past, as a depressingly high percentage of women do, at a minimum she has experienced having her boundaries crossed, sexually or otherwise, or has experienced a man's physical aggression. What she really needs, wants, and craves from you is to feel physically safe.

Emotional, physical, and sexual violence is part of men's historical and generational lineage. It has been a part of men throughout time. What we see so much of in the collective feminine in the world at large right now is a vocal expression that has been accumulating across generations: "We need this to change," "We can't take this anymore," and honestly, "We won't take this anymore." I believe that women in the past felt this, too, but they didn't feel safe and empowered enough to express it. We have reached the point where enough women feel empowered enough and safe enough to express these sentiments despite the fact that violence is still so widespread.

Part of this empowerment is the safety that women have been creating for themselves by banding together, supporting one another, developing their own inner masculine, and building support structures across the globe—and men have created part of that safety, as well. A growing number of men have crossed a certain threshold in their self-development and ownership of their impact. We tend to be less violent than our forebears. We are learning to be more in touch with our bodies and emotions. We are certainly works in progress, but

I do believe that we are increasingly recognizing our effect on women and adjusting accordingly.

Whether we are talking about the #metoo movement or the wide variety of other ways in which women express on social media and beyond, I believe that the underlying expression is simply,

"We just want to feel safe."

I have never physically harmed nor sexually violated a woman, but I have been emotionally violent with women. Many. "Arguing" is a nice way of putting it. "Screaming" would be more accurate. This force inside of me just roaring out at her, cursing at her, being fucking cruel. I have the ability to find where her deepest emotional weaknesses are, and in those moments, I can just twist the knife.

I don't do that anymore. I can't say that I am where I would like to be with such things, but I have made a drastic shift. When I look back, a part of me feels shame—sometimes intense shame. Of course, I attracted women who were battling their demons as much as I was and had their own unhealthy ways of expressing it. It was all too easy to avoid addressing my own fucked-up behaviors because . . . *well, she's no angel, either! If she wasn't so controlling, if she didn't yell at me, if she wasn't so disrespectful, then . . . then . . .* then what? I wouldn't have to raise my voice? I wouldn't be like this? What, am I a completely powerless victim here? She wasn't in my previous relationship or the one before that. I was. Eventually I realized that I was the common denominator in those relationships.

I came to realize that it doesn't matter how a woman—or anyone—interacts with me; she can be toxic as hell, but I am still responsible for my own actions. I know the kind of man that I want to be. If my behavior isn't in alignment with that man, then I am responsible to do whatever I need to do to show up as my Evolved Masculine self, even if that means walking away from the relationship.

I think my fear was that I would be destroyed somehow, that I was losing some semblance of power, that I would be left a weakened shell of myself, so I thought I *had* to fight back. I now know that was never the answer.

My personal experience has led me to believe that pure willpower isn't enough, because I felt powerless to stop myself, and because I wanted this behavior to change long before it did. Once I got triggered, this other version of me would suddenly come out, and he didn't give a fuck—until afterwards. Then the shame would set in.

I have done many things over the years to address my own traumas, and this most likely has played a huge role in why I have walked the path that I have. I went through the sexological bodywork professional training, which also meant receiving the work. I have done a lot of work with dakinis and tantric sexual healers. I have experienced a variety of body work, including getting trained as a bodyworker myself, and I have done different forms of psychological work.

Four things have helped the most:

1. I sought various forms of professional support, from psychotherapy to somatic healing, to release the trauma from my body.

2. I built community around me where I could speak the unspeakable and share the parts of me that I was the most ashamed of.

3. I learned to form a healthier relationship to my anger. Rather than simply hating my anger, I learned to understand what my anger was communicating to me about my boundaries and places where I felt powerless and needed something to change.

4. I fell in love with my infinitely patient wife. Her unconditional love and acceptance, coupled with her ability to speak and hold her boundaries for what she will not tolerate, created a powerful reflection for me to see what needed to change and held me accountable to do the work, all of which made a safe container for me to relax enough to do so.

I believe that a major support for overcoming our most deeply held negative patterns is having a place to talk about these things, having a brotherhood. What I have shared with you here about my verbal and emotional cruelty toward the women I loved . . . *holy shit.* For the vast majority of my life, I didn't say a fucking word to anybody about this. It was my hidden shame. Even as I was rising as a leader and speaker around sexuality, relationship, and men, this was the hidden, shameful part of myself.

The only person who got to know this dark expression of myself was the woman whom I was in love with, the woman I was committed to protecting and taking care of, and whom I wanted to feel the most loved. She was the one whom I wanted to help heal from all her past experiences and what she had experienced with other men. This was the one person in the world who had the worst of me unleashed upon her.

Only recently can I appreciate how isolating it must have been for each of these women to feel like they could not speak to anybody about what they were experiencing with me because they didn't want to negatively affect my reputation. It pains me to realize the ways in which I was simply another version of the very thing that I railed against.

There is a sizable subset of men who seem to actively embrace misogyny and a belief in male superiority. It is easy for those of us who don't fit that category to point fingers and further project our shadow on them, thereby making it easier to avoid addressing the worst of our own behavior.

As I have more successfully wrestled my demons, I notice that I also have a greater compassion for the worst in other men (and women, for that matter). Compassion, though, is not the same as condoning. I do not condone my own worst behaviors, nor do I condone your worst ones, or any other man's. I do wish that other men would have helped hold me accountable. But how could they have done so when I never let any other man know?

Even now, as I write this, I am experiencing intense feelings knowing that it will be read by who knows how many others, strangers and friends alike. At the same time, it feels incredibly freeing.

I have come to relate to these darker impulses as thought viruses or programs that have deeply infected our world. We are born into this world immersed in a variety of messaging, some healthy, some unhealthy. Even if we see and reject these unhealthy thought viruses, they can make their way into our psyches and express themselves in our weakest moments. If we are going to rise up and be the men the world needs and the one she craves, we must commit to doing the deep inner work to root the unhealthy programs out. I believe that starts with coming clean, to talk about this shit, to have other men who can support you and hold you in your weakest moments while reminding you of your strength.

Have there been ways in which the worst of you came out directed at a woman or women? Have you ever made a woman feel unsafe, whether intentionally or unintentionally? How do you know? How does it feel to consider that women might not feel as safe with you as you would have thought?

46.
THE HARMFUL EXPRESSIONS OF THE WOUNDED FEMININE

I spent many years imagining women as being the innocent angels, the good ones. *Men are the problem; women are the victims.* This is certainly a narrative being sold in our culture. Until I was able to see the entirety of what women can be at their very best *and their very worst*—and, of course, everything in between—I was living in the realm of fantasy. I have had direct experiences with the undeniably dark side of women. It is an unpopular but important truth that some women (and men) hold a frame of victim consciousness, most often caused by trauma, that they use to give themselves license to behave in a range of harmful ways. Further, this victimhood allows them to take zero responsibility and therefore zero ownership of their ability to be perpetrators and the ones responsible for causing harm.

I have really struggled around the ways in which I felt punished for the actions of other men, that because I was a nice guy (with poor boundaries) and cared so much and, in that sense, felt safe to them, I became a target for some women to unload their angers and resentments and get their revenge on men. Certain women in my life would sometimes feel justified in behaving shitty toward me because, well, they had been on the receiving end of it from men their whole lives. In that sense, it was their way of getting even, and so I would waffle between being a doormat and being an oppressor.

Maria was a stunningly gorgeous woman who oozed feminine sensuality. Through our relationship, I helped her own the power of her sexuality and to claim it fully without shame. What I didn't anticipate were the ways in which she would use her sexual power to manipulate me and other men, and particularly, to find men who were most susceptible to her feminine allure and use it as a weapon to get what she wanted.

I understand now that this was part of her journey to reclaim her power. After having spent so much of her life feeling disempowered in her relationships and being victimized by men, she had discovered a way to no longer feel like a victim, by making sure that she always had the upper hand. She had me wrapped around her little finger.

While I had a history of emotional violence, Maria would become physically violent. She struck me on four separate occasions, the first of which was while I was driving. *On my birthday.* I know I was probably being an asshole to her. Still, if I had had better boundaries, that would have been the end of our relationship right then and there.

Somebody who strikes their partner once is likely to do it again. While we were at the annual International Conference on Sexuality & Consciousness, where I was appointed to be Master of Ceremonies, things escalated to a new level of mutual toxicity and danger.

In the midst of an argument that morning, she struck me across the face. She lifted her hand back to do it again, and I grabbed her by the wrist to stop the motion. She let out a high-pitched scream. A moment later, the phone rang. It was the front desk of the hotel, asking what was going on and threatening to call the police. I instantly recognized that this was a treacherous situation. Who do you imagine would be the one who would have gotten arrested if the police had come? I told her to leave immediately.

A few months later, while arguing once more, out of nowhere, she struck me across the face yet again. I reflexively yelled at her to stop. *Don't touch me.* She responded by hitting me across my left temple two more times. I grabbed her, trying to wrestle her down. I had a distinct and shocking moment of recognizing that she was using every ounce of her energy to *hurt* me while I was using every ounce of my energy and intention to *not* hurt her.

I realized in that moment how dangerous the situation had become. *She could tear down in a single moment everything I have been working so hard to build. All she has to do is call the police or make the claim of domestic violence, and who is going to be believed? The petite, hundred-pound woman or the freak who calls himself the Erotic Rockstar?*

That was it. I couldn't do this anymore. I released my feeling of responsibility to be the one to help her heal. I had been rationalizing that this was my learning curve around my growth in being a man—that this flavor of feminine reactivity was what I was going to experience until I learned how to strengthen that part of my masculinity.

I had learned that I was simply supposed to be the rock that allowed the feminine storm of her emotions to express in all their wildness. This is what I was, on some level, attempting to do and to be. The story I told myself was that there was something wrong, flawed, or clearly missing about *me* and my masculinity that could not defuse these inflammatory, violent outbursts. I made her unhappiness my fault. I made my inability to calm the feminine storm my fault. It took me a long time to realize that this was not about me but about Maria and *her* trauma imprints, anger, and impulsivity.

Still, the shame I felt around being in an abusive relationship kept me from ever saying a word. Through my exposure to men's online spaces, I knew there were many voices who would point to this situation as evidence that women are the *real* problem—which went against everything I believed in and stood for. I did not want to corroborate the distorted narrative about women, but here I was, having a lived experience of the harmful effects of an abusive woman.

Instead, I just stuffed it inside. I questioned myself again and again: *What did I do wrong? How could I have shown up differently? If I could have just figured out how to be the right kind of man for her, then maybe she could have relaxed and not been so erratic. Then she would have treated me better, and it wouldn't have been so abusive.* Two years later, I found out that during a fight with her boyfriend, she kicked him in the face and broke his nose. As sorry as I was to hear of his injury, there was definitely a certain feeling of vindication in finding this out, as well.

Yes, the sex was great! She was hot as fuck, highly orgasmic, and ran intense feminine sensual energy through her system that would hold me spellbound. The incentives to stay in this relationship were extremely high—and it wasn't my responsibility to fix or heal her. I had reached a place of needing to hold clearer and stronger boundaries of my own.

Of all of my exes, I feel the least resolution with Maria. Even writing this story has been a difficult and emotionally painful process, as it has shown me where I still have unresolved pain. Now, six years later, as much as I am able to take a larger view and hold greater compassion and empathy for her journey, there is also part of me that is still angry and resentful. I have moved through many layers of forgiveness and still feel like there are many to go.

To this day, I sometimes question myself, wondering what I could have done differently, yet as I have come to better understand the generational passing of trauma and my own journey overcoming those patterns, I know that there are elements of her healing that only she is responsible for. I do hope that she has continued to grow and evolve and is able to find and create greater peace in her life.

I know that I have met far too many men (especially on the internet!) who turned cynical and bitter after being hurt by a woman. I think this is particularly pernicious with men who had previously believed in the innocence and purity of women, like I did. When this illusion is shattered, a man is allowed to see her for who she *truly* is: flawed, human, and world-weary. As men, we *must* allow our illusion to be shattered in order to be in a healthy, real relationship with a real human woman.

If you have been hurt by a woman, do whatever you need to do to heal and see women with clean eyes again—or don't, and I hate to say it, but kiss your chances of ever having a healthy relationship goodbye. Even in the worst of dynamics, there are lessons to be learned. Any and every experience you have can be used in service to your evolution.

> Did this story trigger anything inside of you? What fantasies about women do you hold that may interfere with your ability to truly see her in the full scope of her humanity, flaws and all? When have you prioritized a toxic relationship with a woman over your own well-being?

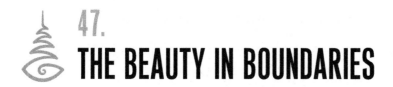

47.
THE BEAUTY IN BOUNDARIES

I came to understand women's boundaries long before I understood my own. Boundaries are a wonderful thing. We use them to keep ourselves safe as we continue to explore. Boundaries can be expanded gracefully or broken with force.

When we look at the wide spectrum of sexual violation, especially with how rampant different forms of sexual trauma are, I have not met a woman who hasn't experienced having her boundaries crossed in some way. What this means is that she may have very good reason to experience fear and contraction during an encounter with you, and it might not have much to do with you. Men can be afraid of women setting boundaries because boundaries can be interpreted as barriers to where they want to go or a signal that they have done something wrong. Worse still, men can interpret women's boundaries as an indication of something wrong with the men themselves at a core level.

I invite you instead to embrace the first boundary she communicates to you, whether it is cued verbally, physically, or energetically. Look for it. Celebrate it. There is something magical that happens when she communicates that first boundary and you respond to it without taking it personally. You neither collapse nor get resentful, but rather, simply honor the boundary: *Oh, okay. Well, let's just play up to the edge of that boundary.* Something in her relaxes; she now knows in that moment that she can trust you with her body and that she can play with you without needing to be on guard.

Something magical tends to happen there, and often, when that happens, the boundary itself moves. Of course, the paradox is that if you are respecting the boundary because you want it to move, it isn't going to work. You need to truly relax into the spaciousness of abundance consciousness. Release the goal. Have patience. Enjoy this moment for this moment's sake.

Boundaries Sometimes Get a Bad Rap

Play like you are a detective trying to uncover where her boundaries are. Explore her boundaries and listen to her body, beyond her words alone. Amplify the pleasure she can experience within the boundaries she sets; she may become curious about what it is like on the other side of the boundary, and move it herself.

Something meaningful happens when she puts up that first boundary and you dance with it just right. You don't ever try to force your way through the boundary, but rather, you stay in your place of ease and fun, and explore those edges. Boundaries can be fluid. They tend to shift in relation to how safe she feels and how much desire she experiences. Show up in a way that you are something she *wants* to be a YES to.

Internal Validation – No Failure, Only Feedback

For you to read her accurately, you cannot take shit personally. This can be a really big one for a lot of men. Rejection can be scary, but regardless of what it feels like, her response to you doesn't validate or invalidate your existence or your worthiness as a man. You must begin with focusing on self-love, internal validation, and a feeling of *enoughness* from within. As you become more sourced from within, you will not require anybody or anything else for you to know your value.

When speaking about sexuality and consent, bringing in feeling of worthiness can seem strange, but I have found that it starts here, because if you aren't self-sourced in finding your validation, everything else starts to become a head game of how to get the validation you seek. This is true whether you seek direct validation from her, from your buddies, your imagined buddies online, or by getting her number, getting that kiss, or getting in her pants in the mistaken belief that that is what makes you a man. All of these head trips cut you out of being present with her in the here and now. What she wants and what will allow her to open to you most is your being present and connected with her.

Think back on your sexual experiences. Have you ever violated a woman's boundary, whether intentionally or unintentionally? How did it make her feel? How did it make you feel? How can you both respect and explore a woman's boundary?

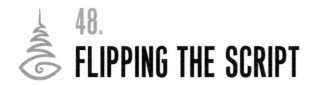

48.
FLIPPING THE SCRIPT

There is a kind of sex she longs for that too many women find elusive. While you may fantasize about your favorite porn position, fucking her anally, or coming across her tits, she fantasizes about overwhelming passion, her heart melting, and her pussy on fire. She yearns to get so turned on in every cell of her body that she explodes into the most powerful orgasm she has ever had the moment she is penetrated with that very first thrust.

Porn teaches a model of sex that, truth be told, is not representative of what most women desire. We have become so impacted, both consciously and unconsciously, by the porn industry that even though we know it is performative, porn sex still has undue influence on how we think and feel about our sex. It literally programs our psyches to think about sex in a linear sequence and therefore to engage with women in a way that is quite frankly not fulfilling to them. Often women are left with a deep longing in their hearts for a quality of sex that they don't often experience outside of their fantasies. The frustration of this chasm has led to an epidemic of sexually unsatisfied women.

As the Erotic Rockstar, I did my best to satisfy *all the women*, but clearly, this will take more than an army of one. All humor aside, this epidemic is the fault of men (with the exception of lesbians, but to my point, they are not usually the sexually unsatisfied ones), and it is our responsibility to transform that sad reality. Doing so is in our best interest, too. Women who have incredible sexual experiences tend to want to have more sex, and most men whom I have met certainly want to experience women's sexual desire more.

So, what do women want? What will set you apart so that her experience with you is unlike her typical experiences with other men? If there is one thing I have learned that completely changes the sexual dynamic with women, it is this:

Flip the script.

Here's the thing: women are used to being sexual gatekeepers. The cultural narrative dictates that the woman has the responsibility to hold things off or give the green light. If she shows even the slightest openness to having sex, she expects him to swoop in and make it happen. He is the ever-driving force toward penetration, while her role is to play defense as the sexual gatekeeper.

Quite often, she is so accustomed to feeling a never-ending onslaught of men's desire for sex that her ability to feel her *own* desire becomes difficult, as she is so busy managing and defending against his insatiable hunger. You have the unique opportunity to learn how to give her the gift of feeling her own desire by learning how to contain and master your own.

The main thing I have learned from working with thousands of men is that for you to be able to flip the script, you must know that you are worthy of a woman's attention. You must believe that a woman could actually want and desire *you*, and that you and your sexuality can be something of real value to her.

You need to make a mental shift from sex being something you get out of a woman to your sexuality being a gift you can share with her. Depending on where you are along your sexual path, this can be a tremendous shift in your understanding of the value of your own sexuality.

In line with this, learning to flip the script requires that you have a mindset of sexual abundance. If you are in a place of scarcity and need, your system is in a state of driving toward *getting*. Flipping the script requires you to override that impulse in order to relax more fully into this moment to connect with what is present for her.

This sense of scarcity has less to do with how long it has been since you last had sex and more to do with your mindset. Coming at women from a place of scarcity will repel them, whereas being in a place of abundance and fullness is highly attractive. I know that this can be challenging, especially if it has been a while since you connected intimately with a woman; however, it is both totally doable and completely worth it.

When I first realized the power of flipping the script in this way, the source of my gratification shifted away from what pleasures I could get out of her to my pleasure becoming sourced in feeling desired *by* her. I learned to evolve my relationship to my own gratification because the positive feedback loop was incredibly rewarding: I would enjoy the little energetic shifts that would occur as she melted and opened further into her own desire.

This is not just a cool trick to get more sex. It is a discipline and a practice—and not always an easy one. Learn to contain and master your own desire so the fires of her passion can be purposefully stoked. There is nothing quite as intoxicating to a woman as a man who can truly hold his sexual energy.

The result of flipping the script is that she has a completely different experience with you than with other men. She gets to the place where her pussy is swollen and soaking wet. It turns the entire dynamic on its head, from her carrying the gatekeeping responsibility to allowing her to surrender to your masculine leadership. Learning to flip the script in this manner is a profound expression of sexual empowerment for men that is also in deep service to her sexual fulfillment. Total win-win.

Do you feel pressure to always be pushing toward sexual intercourse? In what ways (if any) have you been putting your sexual satisfaction before hers from an old-paradigm place of "trying to get sex"? In what ways have you unintentionally been curtailing the full spectrum of her sexual desire and expression? What beliefs would you have to let go of in order to practice flipping the script? Do you believe that you are worthy of being craved for? Do you believe that you and your sexuality could be of value to her?

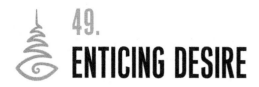

49.
ENTICING DESIRE

When I was young, I learned that the moment a man senses any hint of a woman's desire, he needs to act immediately to drive forward and escalate the situation to greater sexual physicality. As I came to understand feminine sexuality, I stopped approaching sex like that.

She has a desire of her own. You can think of it as a flame inside of her that you can help spark, and then you can fan the flames of that desire. You can draw out that desire, build that sexual tension, and do so in a way that *serves* her desire. I learned to draw out her desire and give her the space to revel in the feeling of that desire. Some refer to this as the art of the tease. I like to think of it as *enticing desire.*

I believe that my path of sexual self-mastery laid the foundation for me to learn how to simply enjoy her desire for its own sake. The more connected I got to my sexual energy, my ability to move that energy, and to simply *be* with that energy, the easier it was for me to let that energy course through my system when I was with her without feeling like I *needed* it to get to any particular end goal. My ESEs taught me how to enjoy the moment-to-moment exploration and process of discovery, which then allow me to take that lens into my interactions with women.

Kirsten had recently broken up with me, and newly single, I had a date for the first time in years. After an evening out, my date, Sabine, and I ended up back at my place. I had put a lot of attention into creating my bachelor pad. There was a succulent, sensual type of flavor to the decor of the space. I put on some sexy, chill electronic music and lit some candles. I was definitely going all out.

I had already made a commitment to myself that I was not going to have sex with Sabine. It was too soon after my breakup, and I simply wasn't ready. I repeated it like a mantra in my mind: *I am not going to have sex with this woman. I am not going to have sex with this woman . . . at least, not tonight.*

Though I hadn't spoken it out loud to her, I had created an internal boundary. I had decided that I would let myself sexually play with her: *I can flirt, I can tease, but I am going to hold this line.* I discovered that there is something powerful in creating this kind of boundary. It turns the dial of sexual tension way up. Though we were kissing, making out, looking into each other's eyes, and exploring each other's bodies with our hands, she never at any moment felt that I was trying to get somewhere—because I had decided that I wasn't going to go there.

The more I didn't push for anything and held that boundary, the more I felt her own desire grow. And grow. And grow. I could feel that turn-on within her. I swear, I noticed and felt that moment at which she decided within herself, *That's it. I'm fucking this man.* I could sense the energetic shift, and I smiled to myself because I knew the decision that I had made. I was feeling her turn on and her ever-increasing craving for me, and I responded to that energy with, "No, not yet. Let's draw out this touch a little bit longer. Let's draw out this kiss a little bit longer. Let's draw out this lick a bit longer." Believing that there was no "there" to get to, I was focused on simply relishing the experience of each moment.

I could feel the fire in her grow brighter and brighter as I held off from fulfilling her desires. Finally, she hit a point at which she said something to me not only with her words but with her tone and energy that I will carry with me for the rest of my life. She succumbed to her desire and cried out, "Please. Please? Please! Fuck me, please. Please, fuck me. Destin, please?! Please fuck me!"

I had never heard a woman say anything like this before, though it wouldn't be the last time a woman literally begged me to fuck her. Having a woman beg you to take and ravish her is a turning point for men in terms of understanding the value they bring to a woman's sexual awakening—and *you* can totally achieve this. I hadn't believed that that kind of dynamic could exist between a woman and a man, and particularly not between a woman and *me*! She could experience her own desire to such a degree and depth that she was quite literally begging.

She continued, and I will admit it . . . I broke.

I swear, I was so committed at the start! However, there were only so many please-fuck-me's I could take. In the moment that I was finally sliding into her,

her eyes shot wide open. I could sense a wave rush through her body as the first of her orgasms took hold.

As you can imagine, this left quite an impression on me. It's one thing for a woman to let me "have my way" with her and another for her burning desire to be so bright that she wants it, needs it, craves it, and literally begs for it. This quickly became my new biggest turn-on and my new favorite game to play. I learned to flip the script and entice *her* desire.

I started to take this approach into every interaction and sexual experience that I had with a woman, especially when we were connecting for the first time. I wanted to create that kind of energy and dynamic again. I wanted to feel her desire. I never again wanted to feel like a woman was letting me through her defenses. No, I was determined to put my focus on learning how to make this my new normal. I would master the art of sparking her desire and then drawing it out from her until she was the one leaning in, eagerly waiting for me to say OK.

If you are solely focused on being the driving force toward the sex, you can't build the sexual tension; this is when she becomes a gatekeeper. If she feels your desire and your "push" energy moving beyond where she is at, then she has one of two options. She can just let it happen before she is fully ready, or she can defend against it, push against it. Move it aside, or make up an excuse and say she has to go.

In the time since that night with Sabine, I have gotten better at all aspects of this *enticing desire* game, including my ability to hold my own desires and boundaries. For me to experience true sexual self-mastery, I needed to learn how to successfully hold my boundary even in the face of such enticement on her part. Sovereignty of my own body and sexuality means being able to stick to my *no* if it doesn't feel in alignment and to not let my sexual turn-on overrule my conscious will. That said, I like to believe that succumbing to her desire that night actually did serve the greater good, given where that moment eventually led me.

Are you normally the one who pulls off her clothes first? Are you typically the one who progresses the sexual encounter toward intercourse? How can you entice her desire? Draw out her passion while remaining immersed and present in the moment. Challenge yourself to get her to crave you, even beg you for more.

50.
SEXUAL ATTUNEMENT AND CONSENT

After my relationship with Anjali, I had seemingly opened Pandora's box. By this time I was in college, and I had somehow become the guy with whom women shared their appalling stories of rape, sexual violation, and harassment. Once started, it just never stopped. I can't tell you how many women's stories I have heard, often through tears as I held their hands. Frequently, if I wasn't the first person she had told, I was certainly the first *man* she had told.

Over the next decade and change, I came to eye other men with suspicion and distrust. Step by step (and unintentionally), I stopped making male friends and came to populate my life with women as friends, roommates, bosses, and lovers.

From this deep immersion with women, I came to understand things that I otherwise would never have known. The sheer number of women who have had their will overpowered by men lustful for sex or a feeling of power was shocking to me, and wildly disturbing.

What took me longer to understand, though, was that some women—especially those who have experienced trauma—have a hard time saying no even when they want to. She may go along with sex with a man because she felt intimidated by him, or didn't want to disappoint him, or otherwise didn't know how to say no. However, these experiences, too, often have a lasting negative impact on her, how she experiences men moving forward, and how easy or difficult it is for her to trust men.

Fuck. I do not want to leave that kind of mark on a woman. I do not want to be that guy. I can't let that be me. I think this is the real reason why I developed my unusual approach to creating intimacy with women: it minimized any likelihood that I would unintentionally violate her. It felt both powerful *and safe.*

I have come to see that while there are indeed men who simply have malicious intent, there are many more men who inadvertently commit "consent violations" without intention and are sometimes even completely unaware that they have. However, impact always trumps intention, so whether or not a man is aware of it, real harm may be done.

Too many of us were raised on shitty, outdated scripts of how we are "supposed to" engage with women. Compound this with poor-to-mediocre attunement, and harm is waiting to happen.

The #metoo movement has been a giant mirror for us as men, reflecting how we have received flawed programming when it comes to sex and women, and particularly, how that flawed programming has caused a tremendous amount of harm, which we are only now beginning to confront. #Metoo is an opportunity that challenges men to develop greater emotional intelligence, of which sexual attunement is an organic extension. It has forced a reorganization of power dynamics between men and women in the bedroom and beyond. The old paradigm dynamic (as described in chapter 49, "Enticing Desire") of driving force (him) and gatekeeper (her) is no longer viable, and instead, we are being asked to play a better game.

We do not, however, have to make the male sexual experience smaller or more contracted. Not only would that suck for us, but women *do not* want tentative men who do not know how or are afraid to create intense sexual containers and experiences for them. They want men who can stand in their power *and* have developed sexual attunement *so that* they can have a wide range of sexual adventures together.

Sexual attunement is seeing, hearing, and feeling her, tuning in and noticing her experience moment by moment, and making micro-adjustments along the way.

Historically, men have had a substandard attunement to women's desires and boundaries. The writing is on the wall: *those days are over*. Instead of meeting this new playing field with frustration, confusion, or denial, we have a significant opportunity available to us within this evolving social landscape. This is not necessarily complicated, but it does require a re-envisioning of who you are as a sexual being.

Most people, men and women, would strongly benefit by learning to communicate more clearly about their desires, fears, and boundaries when it comes to sexual intimacy. If there was ever a time to dial this in, it is now. The stakes are high. Women are more aware than ever before of the prevalence of sexual assault, and men are more concerned than ever about doing something that will either cause harm or get themselves into trouble. This is why sexual attunement is so important. We are in the midst of a serious sexual trauma crisis, and I believe that sexual attunement is a key part of the solution.

When it comes to sexual attunement, start with the most obvious, and as you become more attuned, you can sink into the ever-more-subtle awarenesses. We start with verbal communication. Build the practice of speaking your desire and what you want to do. Use your words to draw out a clear yes or no from the woman you are engaging with.

When in doubt about her experience or desire, *ask her*. Verbal and nonverbal communication can be used in concert—in fact, I would argue that they always are. Getting verbal consent does not need to be disruptive or unsexy; it can be quite the opposite. You can use verbal communication to ask for consent in a seductive and explicit manner, creating even more turn-on between you and your partner in the process. How she responds to you is less about your choice of words and more about the energy you hold and project.

The key skills to develop are as follows:

1. Express your desire,

2. in an inviting and seductive manner,

3. with total respect for her ability to make choices of what she does and does not want to do,

4. while remaining unattached to the outcome.

Sexual attunement is a constant conversation of consent and desire that sometimes takes place verbally and often does not. It is said that 60 to 70 percent of communication is nonverbal, so she is in continuous communication with you. In Part III, "Sexual Self-Mastery," you learned to pay attention to the subtleties in your body that you may never noticed before. That process will also train your system so that you will have an easier time noticing subtleties in *her* that you have likely not noticed previously.

Masculine sensitivity is the very foundation of sexual attunement, yet the old cultural narrative has regarded men's sensitivity as both feminine and a weakness. This distorted understanding leads many men to feel ashamed of their own sensitivity, as they do not yet understand that their sensitivity is directly proportional to their ability to attune to their lover's body and what she truly desires.

Growing up, I was always told that I was too sensitive. However, my sensitivity was at the root of the Erotic Rockstar's ability to create mind-blowing sexual experiences for both my lovers and myself. Your sensitivity can be developed into a superpower and can bring forth an incredible masculine sexual potency.

The attunement process may be highly confronting for you because it requires that you get out of your head about what you think you are "supposed" to do. There is no preset playbook for what part of her body to touch and when in order to "get a woman to have sex" with you; it is, in fact, the opposite. Just get out of your head and learn to become fully present. Drop into your five senses and tune in to the subtleties of what is happening moment by moment so you can respond accordingly. The idea of not thinking about what to do may well be a massive mindfuck for you, yet only through your dropped-in presence will you be able to truly tune in to the subtleties of what is happening in her body.

Tune in to all of the micro-communications in her body language. With every look, with every touch, with every kiss, her body will respond in some way. It may be with direct, overt movements or with subtle micro-movements, the slight little tensions or relaxations of the body that most people completely miss but that are there. If you start to pay attention to these subtleties, to both watch and feel for them, you will begin to notice the constant communication that occurs.

Begin to notice that slight little movement in her posture, a shift in the look in her eyes, the changes in her breath, and any movement that suggests her body is closing—or where her body language is opening.

Imagine being so tuned in to her that you are aware of her every inhale and exhale. By matching her breath, you can get a sense of what it feels like to be in her body. Your energetic and neurological systems start to align with hers when you breathe in time together. The practices you began working with in Part III to build a relationship with your own breath will make it easier for you to connect to the rhythm of her breathing.

By paying attention to her micro-movements, you can respond and redirect your energy before she even has the opportunity to say something. She will start to feel like you are able to read her mind, as before she even opens her mouth to communicate to you verbally, you will have already noticed and started to course-correct.

Instead of reacting to any little contraction of hers with collapse and apology, practice listening for the deeper communication, and gently explore redirecting your approach. The following is a real-life scenario a client described to me about a recent experience of his: He and a woman were deep in make-out mode. He goes to lift her dress. She says, "Not yet." He took it personally and made it about him, his performance, and his worthiness as a man. She felt his sudden shutdown and also drew back. Soon after, their date ended, and she went home. After she left, he bounced back and forth between beating himself up and telling himself stories about how he wasn't really that into her anyway in an effort to protect his ego before she could reject his request for another date.

This all-too-common situation perfectly highlights why developing sexual attunement is so valuable. Her "not yet" may have been a request for him to slow down or an invitation for him to turn her on more before her dress came off. It could have been an opportunity for him to refine his process of attuning to her before he made her "not yet" into a judgment about him.

And maybe, just maybe, that "not yet" really meant that she wasn't ready to go there at all during this date. Sometimes, continuing to entice her desire simply may not be about a single date. Giving space and being responsive yet nonreactive to her boundary increases the likelihood that she will go home and wonder what if: What if she hadn't put up that boundary? What if she had let herself go further? What would that experience have been like? Her longing and being in a space of suspended desire is certainly a better outcome than her going home feeling regret, and it certainly creates a greater chance of having that next date.

The knife's edge that is presented to us as men is in finding where that line is between her desire to be further opened and a hard no. However, you cannot accurately learn to differentiate the two until you are able to stay clear, present, and curious, and neither in your anxiety about doing the wrong thing nor so focused on what you want that you aren't truly paying attention to her.

Another key piece in the process of guiding and leading a woman sexually is pacing. This is an area where men tend to shoot themselves in the foot. Have you ever had that experience with a woman where she seemed to want the same thing you did and everything seemed to be moving along well, but then suddenly she closed down and got more distant? Or maybe she continued to go along with things, but you noticed that she wasn't as enthusiastic anymore. Well, there is a good chance that you were trying to get there faster than she was opening. Too many men end up getting so lost in their own desires that they don't listen or attune to her body, her responses, and her *pacing*. Don't be so focused on your imagined goal that you leave her behind. Her body will contract, and next thing you know, she says, "I have to go"—or worse, she will continue to go along with things and then leave feeling disrespected or violated, or both.

Going slow sometimes means going half your normal speed of touch, and then half that, and then half that still. Sometimes, though, it just means slowing it down 10 percent; sometimes even 1 percent slower can make all the difference. This is why it is key to tune in, pay close attention, and listen to the shifts in her body language, breathing patterns, and sounds.

Women tend to be better than men at picking up on body language. I believe this is because so many men live in their heads, analyzing the situation, instead of being in their bodies and fully experiencing the situation. The deeper you are in your own body, the easier it is to feel what is going on for you, and therefore, the easier it will be for you to feel what is going on for her.

The body has mirror neurons that fire off in response to the neurons that light up in another person's body. This is why you can experience such rich feeling and emotion while watching a movie and why you can watch somebody perform a task and learn to do it yourself. You can learn to get a sense of what is going on in her body through a combination of paying close attention to the subtleties in her and tuning in to and feeling the little shifts in your own body.

One of the many gifts that Kirsten left me with was a love of playing with my balls—a four-inch acrylic crystal ball and a two-and-a-half-inch one, to be exact. Contact juggling, a circus talent of hers that I also made my own. I considered it another of my dojos. I could be in the midst of a thousand partygoers with strobe lights flashing and bass music blaring, and it was just me and my ball. I would pour the fullness of my attention into this little crystal ball, and everything else would disappear. It taught me to focus in, with fine-tuned attention, to how the slightest movement created a response in this external object.

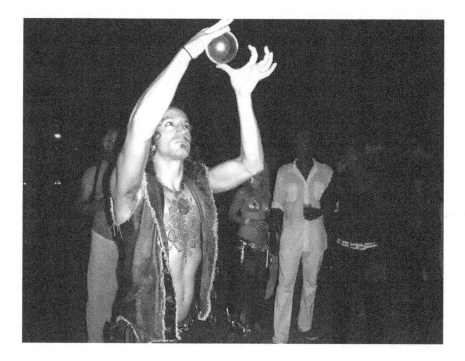

I learned to treat sex and a lover's body the same way. I learned to be so keenly focused that everything outside of her would fade into the background. All thoughts, worries, concerns, and fantasies were put on pause. I learned to tune in to her body and feel for the most subtle of sensations and movements. Just as she would start to move, before she would even realize she was moving, I would be right there, moving in time with her.

If my fingers were inside of her, then all of my attention and awareness were on my hand and in her body. This means that as I was feeling her vaginal musculature around my fingers, I was also tuned in to the flow of energy within, and the flow of her breath, and the sounds that she made. As she moved, my hand moved in time with her. Just as I could play the instrument of the glass ball, where the slightest movements of my hands and fingers created exponential magic, I could also tune in to my lover's body so that the slightest of movements carried profound energetic information. When you touch a woman, you don't always have to do intense finger banging (though that has its place); you can also make the tiniest of motions.

You may notice that composers do not simply create their symphonies entirely in fortissimo. The intensity is much more effective when it can be used in contrast. You can learn to play with the subtlest of subtlety as well as the most intense of intensities, and every flavor in between. It is all available to you, and you can bring it all to her.

She can learn to be attuned to feeling your micro-movements just as you can tune in to how her body responds to these little sensations and small movements. This level of awareness is something to cultivate over time. The more attention you give to attuning to your lover, day by day and experience by experience, the more you will grow your ability to feel and transmit subtle sexual sensations.

What I love about sexual attunement is that its development is a key to creating greater emotional and physical safety for women, while also actively allowing men to tap in to a deeper state of presence and power. The more you are able to attune to your lover's body, the more incredible and wildly pleasurable sexual experiences you will be able to create for you both.

How have you approached women you have been attracted to in the past? Have you come across as too intense? Have you come across as too timid? How did she respond? Be bold, yet pay close attention to her feedback, both verbal and nonverbal. What can you become aware of that you had never noticed before?

51.
ALL MEN ARE SEXUAL HEALERS

About a decade ago, for one of my first podcast appearances, I was a guest on "Embodying Masculine Desire," featuring host Robert Allen. Robert was a colleague of mine who created and facilitated a workshop with the startling (to me) title: "All Men Are Sexual Healers." When I first heard this title, my whole system contracted in confusion and defiance. *What does he mean, "all men are sexual healers"? Doesn't he know that men are THE reason why sexual healing is necessary in the first place? Besides, becoming a sexual healer is a path—and a long, complex, and deeply confronting one, at that. It is an intense commitment. And hey, I've put all this work in to become a "real" sexual healer, so how can you diminish me like that and say that "all men are sexual healers"?* (My ego was clearly getting the better of me.)

It is now a decade later, and I am *still* grappling with the statement "All men are sexual healers." Only now am I able to see the beauty in it. In North America and beyond, we are reckoning with just how widespread sexual trauma is. Millions of women have raised their hands to say #metoo, and we know that there are millions more who have yet to find the courage to share their stories of sexual abuse and trauma.

As men on an intentional evolutionary path, we have the opportunity to look at ourselves, our ways of relating to women and sex, our belief systems, and of course, our own behavior. We have the opportunity—and ultimately, the responsibility—to not only not be another man who causes her harm, but to be an active part of her sexual healing. As I write these words, I am aware that they make a bold statement—men have the opportunity and the responsibility to be *an active part of her sexual healing*. What could this possibly even look like?

As with all things, it begins with you. Becoming a man with the capacity to heal through his sex requires that you radically address your own sexual healing. When I use the word *healing*, I simply mean becoming more whole.

There is something profoundly impactful and deeply healing for a woman about being penetrated by a man with a strong and loving connection between his heart and his cock, when he shows up fully present, fully loving, fully in his desire and its expression, and is deeply attuned to her, her body, her autonomy, her wants and needs, her yes and her no.

In my admittedly extravagant seven-year stint of sexcapades, I discovered that there is something profoundly healing for a woman who has had her boundaries breached to be with a man who is *fully* committed to honoring her needs—*and her desires*. I came to understand that each of these aspects of women—their need for safety (communicated as boundaries) *and* their desire for pleasure—are vitally meaningful within an erotic encounter. I have learned that there is an inherently healing effect for a woman to experience a man who is fully present and committed to understanding her boundaries, and who can do so without sacrificing the animal within and his ability to experience and create ravenous desire.

I learned how to help women feel seen, heard, and felt. It was my intention that she understand at the core of her being that *all* of who she is matters; her wants and desires, her fears and concerns all matter. Her boundaries matter. Her body and her sexuality are hers to do with as she chooses, *how she chooses*. She can say no as she chooses and express herself and her sexuality as wildly as she chooses, and I will support and celebrate her emergence into her fullness and power.

To my dismay and growing concern, I had the unfortunate honor of learning just how rare it is for women to interact sexually with a man who carries this frame and intention. In a more positive light, I have also witnessed how deeply freeing it feels when she is seen and unconditionally accepted as she is and for all that she is.

When she is held in a container within which her autonomy is sacrosanct, a level of safety is created that she may have been yearning for her whole life. When she no longer feels like she has to conform to a man's preconceived notions and fantasies of what her sexuality is *supposed* to be, the true gift of her authentic sexual expression begins to unfold and blossom.

A great misconception in the world of dating and discussions around men and women is the notion that her sexuality and desire need to be coaxed out of her. This is simply not true. The responsibility lies with you to create the right conditions for her sex and desire to open to you. Sex is not something that is "gotten"; it is something that is *co-created*. I learned to create containers, or *energetic bubbles*, around the two of us, with the intention of inviting her in to safely explore her sexuality. By and large, women *want* to explore their sexuality and deepen their knowing of their own bodies and their own pleasure. However, too often, they learned early in their sexual development that they need to be on guard with men.

While he learns that his role is to constantly escalate romantic encounters toward the end goal of sex, she learns to play defense. So long as she is in a defensive role, she cannot relax. If she is not relaxed, then she is not feeling good on some level. If she is not relaxed and feeling good, her curiosity cannot come out to play.

Sexual self-mastery teaches you how to hold and contain your sexual energy. This way, you can feel the fullness of your desire and allow it to emanate out from you in a way that is tangible and felt by her, and yet—and this is a critical distinction—*you are the keeper and the master of your desire*. You are not enslaved to your desire, which is the lived experience of so many men who are not exposed to teachings about their sex.

You achieve mastery when you can feel the desire and be at full conscious choice as to what you do with that desire. As I mastered this, my lovers were turned on by my desire while simultaneously feeling safe through my ability to remain conscious and connected with my own desire. My desire is *mine*. I can choose to share it with my lovers in parallel with being fully responsible for creating the right conditions for her to receive it in a way that serves her desire *and* her safety.

There are parts of my journey as the Erotic Rockstar that are difficult for me to talk about. One such aspect is my ego. Despite my good intentions and the intense investments I made to stay in integrity, there were times when I definitely allowed my ego to get carried away. Part of me felt like I had developed erotic superpowers.

To throw down in full transparency, there was an abundance of women longing for what I had in part because of, well, my own unique magic, but also because there was a dire lack of men who had consciously created themselves as lovers. There was a point on my path at which I was receiving so much positive feedback, validation, and straight-up sexual reward from women that I had the admittedly bloated idea that I could be this awesome and healing lover for *all* the women. But this is the saving grace about being committed to a personal spiritual path: you get your ass kicked, and as a result, you grow.

I came to see things that I hadn't seen before. After being sex-drunk for several years, I slowly sobered up and came to realize that, yes, there was indeed something I could open up and fulfill for many women: a deeply held desire to be wildly ravished *and* wildly attuned to at their deepest feminine essence; however, there was something else, something deeper she was yearning for that I could not meet. It wasn't until I was ready to have that something in myself be met that I could understand what it was that I couldn't meet in her.

I realized that this is what Robert Allen was referring to when he said all men are sexual healers. For our culture to truly heal and for this massive distrust and division between men and women to reconcile, men need to not only stop doing shitty things and checking their brothers to stop doing shitty things, though that is a big part of it; they also need to start being an active part of the sexual healing.

You have the capability for your sex to have a healing capacity, but only if you choose to. It is a big responsibility, and not something to take lightly. Playing at this level requires you to go through a major evolution. A woman's heart and body are on the line here, a woman who may already carry trauma.

You can't just look at women as broken little birds whom you have to come in and save, either. I have gone that route, and it backfired horrendously. This approach always starts off great; however, it builds a power dynamic into the relationship that she will eventually have to rebel against. She is on her own path to discover herself and her empowerment. The rescuer dynamic requires a victim, so for her to fully reclaim her power, she will ultimately have to reject you.

I was hesitant to write this chapter because I have seen the problems that can arise from men calling themselves sexual healers and then using that label to prey upon unsuspecting women in search of their own healing. However, in this era, with so much attention on the ways in which male sexuality can (and does) harm, I believe it is important to know that there is a way you can align your sexuality so that it can be a gift that heals. The minute you use your sexual healing capacity as a line or a tool to get her into bed with you is the moment you set things up to create unintentional harm.

This change requires an identity-level shift. If you are tired of being seen as the problem, then be an active part of the solution. This requires a willingness to be acutely responsible for your sexuality. It doesn't mean simply not causing direct harm. It means owning the good you can impart from your sex by bringing your sexuality into alignment with the whole of who you are, mind, body, and spirit. It means showing up clearly, in your body, fully present with her, fully connected, seeing her. It means having something to offer and share from the gift of your sexuality instead of simply seeking what you can get. It means learning to deeply listen and become sexually attuned to the little shifts and changes that occur in her body, where her yeses are, and where her noes are expressed. And it means mastering the magic formula of helping her feel safe and turned on in the right proportions.

Do this, and your sexuality will be a gift that opens her, a gift that heals her and helps her feel more whole. It will be a gift that helps her forgive and trust in men and the masculine, a gift that helps her blossom more fully into the truth of who she is and the woman she is capable of becoming. In making this identity shift, she will open you in return.

Could your sexuality be a healing force? What would have to shift in how you relate to women and yourself for your sexuality to be a gift that heals? What impact do you believe engaging with your sex as a healing force would have on YOU?

52.
DEVOTION TO THE FEMININE

In my process of learning to distinguish the difference between women and the feminine, I fell in love with both. I fell in love with women and the incredible array of expressions they have, including the wide spectrum of ways that different women carry and express the interplay of the feminine and masculine aspects within themselves.

I also fell in love with the feminine itself. I developed a fascination for truly understanding and knowing this mysterious energetic force. I created a personification of feminine energy in my mind's eye of the cosmic *Woman*, who contains and includes all women.

If the ineffable nature of divinity itself consists of both masculine and feminine in equal balance, and the God that I was raised on was specifically male, then that meant there was a whole other side of divine expression I was completely unfamiliar with. I encountered Her through the incredible women who graced my life, each of whom enchanted me in her own unique way.

I fell in love with the core essence energy that I could find and get to know in each woman I have loved. There were multiple driving forces behind my promiscuity as the Erotic Rockstar, but one that was least understood by others was my desire to sample all the different fractals of Her. Through diversity, I could see Her kaleidoscopically from many different angles, each one helping me to understand Her more fully. Making love to her allowed me to see Her most intimately. With each successive woman, I gathered another piece of the puzzle so I could put together a more complete picture of who She really is.

Allow yourself to be fascinated by her, whether Woman with a capital W or the specific woman in your life. Who is she? How does she tick? How does she experience this world? Allow yourself to become fascinated with every little thing—this is what it is to be fascinated. Every little thing inspires a curiosity to come alive in you.

Fascination creates intimacy. Think of something you are fascinated by or seriously into: a particular musical genre, cars, sport, photography, and so on. As a result of your fascination with that subject or activity, you know a thousand subtle aspects and details about it. This is what is possible if you allow and stoke the fires of your fascination with this thing we call *the feminine*. Your fascination will automatically lead you to greater awareness and understanding. It is through fascination that you can remain the perpetual student and retain what Buddhism refers to as the *beginner's mind*. From a place of fascination comes a desire to know more and understand on a deeper level while recognizing that, in very real ways, there is always more to learn.

It was from this level of fascination that I began to pay close attention to her breath, her sounds, her words, her body language, and the micro-tensing and relaxation of her musculature. I came to develop an incredible sensitivity, noticing ever-greater levels of subtlety that most people never pick up on. This, though, is the power of devotion: continually giving effort and attention in this direction and allowing myself to follow the fascination over time.

Seduction is an act of devotion when done right, and devotion itself can be quite seductive. Women desire to feel adored, even worshiped, by a man. The man she craves is unafraid of adoring and worshiping her instead of fearing this would weaken him in some way. He can do so from his strength and center, not from subservience but from power. With that, she wants to be inspired to adore and worship him, as well, instead of feeling pressured or obligated.

Serving her in this way is not supplication but rather is sourced from a place of fullness within. Being in your gifts, your power, and your overflow while being in service to her will bring you joy and satisfaction. Whether she is your committed partner, a lover, or a passing stranger, you can still be in service to her and her path. You can still be in service to her self-discovery process, growth, and further opening. Paradoxically, your unconditional adoration will most inspire her desire to pour forth her own adoration of you.

I relate to adoration, worship, and devotion as practices. We are always in practice. Everything we do is practice. A lot of us have learned to hold back and cut off from parts of ourselves, showing up as less than because we don't want to give all of ourselves until we meet that one deserving person. Quite honestly, though, we do ourselves a disservice when we hold back.

I created a video product for couples, called the "Gift of Puja," with a colleague of mine, Monique Darling. Together, we led a group of two hundred men and women through a set of experiences, playing with adoration, devotion, and worship as practices for their own sake.

As the participants took turns exploring these practices with different partners, they discovered the power of opening their heart and pouring love for no reason at all into the human being who was before them, even if they were a total stranger. How does this apply to you? You may not know their name, they may never do anything for you in return, and you may never see them again, yet you have the opportunity to practice giving for the sake of giving. Loving for the sake of loving. Love, after all, is a practice, one most of us could use more practice in.

Adoration, worship, and devotion are all forms of giving fully. They are acts of service and have an unconditional quality to them. However, there are two primary pitfalls in the domain of giving. The first one is giving from a state of depletion or emptiness, which can lead to resentment. The second is giving with the hope of getting. Adoring someone because you want something from them is not adoration, it is manipulation.

If you want to be an extraordinary Evolved Masculine lover, you need to learn how to give unconditionally, and in order to do that with any sustainability, you have to be an extraordinary receiver so that you can be fulfilled, whole, and giving from a cup that is overflowing.

Find that place of giving that is not just for your lover but also for you to have the experience of adoring, devotion, and showing up fully. Being in this type of practice helps you to open further to your own greatness and capacity. One of the reasons why I am able to show up for and give to my wife as fully as I do is because I practiced. I practiced with all my partners and my casual lovers before her. *How much of myself can I give?*

I had to learn how to give myself fully while taking care of myself and not overstepping my boundaries. *What can I give that I can give unconditionally?* Once you give conditionally, you overstep what you should be giving. My practice within that boundary has been to continue to expand how much I can give unconditionally, for the sheer joy of giving itself.

In general, our larger culture relates to surrender as a form of weakness. Surrender in this context means giving up, quitting, or allowing yourself to be conquered. However, there is another definition of surrender that is potent and beautiful: the act of just letting go, releasing control, taking all that you have been holding on to—your body, your beliefs, your sense of reality—and releasing, surrendering to your lover, to life, and to this moment. While the opportunity to surrender sounds like an oxymoron, it can be one of the most profound gifts you have to offer her.

Many women today feel like they have to push, struggle, be in defensive mode, and be in their masculine to make their way in a man's world. You can learn to create an environment in which a woman feels safe and held, with enough trust in you to let go completely, to surrender her body and being fully, to allow the force of divinity itself to flood through her body. It is a powerful act and a beautiful sight to behold.

Responsibly creating the space of trust, safety, and desire for her to be able surrender is a gift that you have to offer her. Her surrender is itself a gift that she has to offer you. There is something about a turned-on, wildly expressed woman in the throes of sexual surrender that has the power to blast open a man in ways that cannot be expressed with words alone.

My exploration of tantra led me to approach relationship as a spiritual path and practice.

If each of us is a physical manifestation of the divine itself,
then she is the altar at which I pray.

— Destin Gerek

So get on your knees and pray.

Kneel before her. Look up at her with total love, adoration, and devotion in your eyes. Explore her body with your eyes, your hands, your nostrils, and your tongue. Listen to her sounds—her moans of pleasure, even the sound of each inhalation and exhalation.

Drink her in with your eyes. In a world where a woman is often looked at as a piece of meat, see her as a work of art, a masterpiece in her own right; every perceived flaw, perfectly designed for her unique soul's journey of growth and evolution. Every imperfect way in which she interacts with you is a perfect reflection for you to see yourself, your reactions, and your own areas of growth.

Touch her body as if you were a blind man reading braille, as if, through your touch, you are reading her the beauty of her body, helping her to see it as if for the first time, through the love that pours through your fingertips.

Explore every freckle and beauty mark, every fold of tissue and wrinkle in her skin, the shifts in skin tone from one area to another. As you trace the contours of her body, pay close attention. How is she responding? Pay attention to her sounds, the changes in her breathing, the way she arches and moves her body.

To be an Evolved Masculine lover is to play a game of being in a state of constant exploration. What excites her? What turns her on? How does her sexual energy tend to move through her body? How can you engage with that energy? Learn to play her body like an instrument. What movements strike which chords? What combinations of chords play a melody? How long do you hold each note? How do you intentionally play with the spaces between the notes?

How do you make a woman feel met physically, emotionally, intellectually, sexually, spiritually, whether it is to build a life with her or to spend just a night? You can have a casual experience with somebody and still care. You can still show up fully, give of yourself, and want and desire the very best for this person. Show up in such a way that your sexual connection itself is opening, expansive, and a growth experience for everybody involved. The starting point to doing so is to simply hold the intention.

As you understand by now, the feminine is multidimensional; it includes more than the human embodiment of woman. As the giver and sustainer of life, Earth itself has historically been related to as feminine (as exemplified through the use of the phrase "Mother Earth"). Our planet is in serious crisis because of a lack of reverence, and it is only by devotion to the feminine through how we treat the Earth that we can save ourselves from an otherwise certain extinction. In this sense, devotion to the feminine is both long overdue and has hit a point in which it is simply a necessity.

I have come to think of my work as an expression of my devotion to the feminine through service to men and the masculine. As such, there have been countless times in which a woman has come up to me simply to express her gratitude for the work I do with men. Without my saying anything about it, some women see right away that supporting men on this path serves both men and women, just as your commitment to this path will serve both you personally and any and all women you connect with.

In my Erotic Rockstar years, I was primarily focused on what I could learn about devotion to the feminine through a wide variety of women. As I deepened into my Evolved Masculine path, I eventually came to focus on learning about the feminine primarily through an ever-deepening devotion within my commitment to one woman across years: my wife. Devotion is what calls me to continue to show up, even in the most difficult moments. Devotion is why I make personal sacrifices to ensure that the people I care for have what they need. Devotion is what leads me to continually confront the most uncomfortable parts of myself, which I may otherwise wish to avoid, as my devotion keeps me committed to being the very best man I can be, including how I choose to show up for the ones I love. Through this devotion to her/Her, I am continually inspired and challenged to rise up and become more than I had ever imagined I was capable of. It is your devotion to the feminine that is the key to realizing and embodying your most Evolved Masculine self.

> What you continually dedicate your time, energy, and attention to is the best indicator of your devotion. What have you been devoted to? Are these the things that most serve you in becoming the man you desire to be? Do you believe that you can be someone whom a woman would willingly sexually surrender to? How do you express devotion?

PART 5
THE PATH CONTINUES

53.
LEARNING TO LOVE: THE STORY OF ELIE

In 2003, at twenty-five years old, I was in a psychedelic trance music and clothing store on Haight Street in San Francisco, when in walked this Japanese fashionista raver girl. I immediately felt something light up inside of me. A moment later, I saw her boyfriend walk in right behind her. Disappointed, I decided, *Fuck it,* and walked over to introduce myself to both of them. This was the moment I met Elie. Over the next few months, Elie and I built a friendship and continued to bond. We both felt a strong chemistry between us right from the beginning. When her boyfriend flew back to Japan, she and I did our best to honor the boundaries of her relationship while continuing to explore our deepening friendship.

I remember one evening, hanging out at her place, listening to music, smoking a spliff, and drinking Japanese tea. There came a moment when our eyes locked. Though neither of us knew anything about tantra, we inadvertently slipped into a highly tantric experience during which everything else faded into the background and then disappeared as we became lost in each other's eyes. I remember lightly stroking her cheek and feeling an electric charge pass between us through my touch.

Out of respect for her boyfriend, we agreed to not kiss, yet what we shared that night was extraordinarily intimate and powerful. We were intoxicated in each other's presence, leaning as close as we could without crossing the "no kissing" boundary, the energy swelling and building between us. This potent sensual energy felt as if it were filling my entire being while she was experiencing the same. More than once I said, "I have to go" or she whispered, "You should probably go," and yet we couldn't take our eyes off one another or break the gaze. Our fingers started to caress each other's hair. We brought our cheeks up against one another so that they were millimeters apart, not quite touching and yet able to feel one another. I distinctly remember the feeling of my hair standing up on the back of my neck, my body flush with so much sensation and turn-on coursing through our connection.

After that special night, we backed off of our sensual interactions and settled into a platonic relationship. Despite the ever-present intensity of what Elie always called our "special friendship," the timing to get together was never right. By the time Elie broke up with her boyfriend, I was with Kirsten. My relationship with Kirsten ended just as Elie was preparing to move back to Japan.

She spent her last night in the United States at my place, and at long last, we had sex together for the first time, four years after that initial meeting and hours before she took off to move halfway across the world. In life, there is a unique sort of electricity that runs through nights like these.

And then she was gone.

Five years later, I took a VIP client to Kyoto for a ten-day spiritual/sexual transformational coaching adventure. After years apart, Elie joined me, along with my client, for our last two days. As I witnessed her having a profound impact on my client's transformational journey, I quickly discovered the unique spiritual and energetic talents that she had cultivated in our time apart. After he left, Elie and I spent a week together with nothing holding us back. We had been waiting nine years for this moment. We took full advantage of our newfound freedom and had an intense sexual interlude with one another. All too quickly, my time in Japan ended, and I flew off to meet a different client for an adventure in Nepal.

Little did I know that that week together activated something and set in motion a destiny that I could never have predicted. I had accepted that this was just another example of how our timing was never right: she was in the middle of a five-year discipleship with an advanced spiritual teacher, during which she was living half-time in the jungle of a small island in the Philippines. Meanwhile, I was still deep in my Erotic Rockstar lifestyle, halfway around the world in California.

A year and a half later, Elie visited me in California, and it quickly became clear that she might be what I had been searching for. I was thirty-five years old, six months out of my toxic relationship with Maria, and my mother had just passed away. I was feeling a deep and rapidly increasing yearning for a family of my own.

The whole first year of my relationship with Elie was a bit challenging for me. She was neither a stripper nor a model, which I had been nearly exclusively dating in the ten preceding years. If I was a sexually focused being with a strong spiritual side, Elie was a spiritually focused being with a strong sexual side.

Some part of me felt like something was missing, but I couldn't put my finger on what it was. Our relationship felt so different from others I had had. *Something's weird. Something's missing.* I started to realize that what was missing was all the unnecessary drama, the constant turbulence, and the emotional roller coaster. I had finally landed in a healthy and stable relationship, and while we still had challenges ahead and likely still do, I knew that I had found what I had been looking for.

In 2017, we married. We now have a beautiful baby girl, and I experience more joy and laughter in my life each day than I used to experience in a year. My professional effectiveness and the success of my business have soared since I committed to Elie. This relationship is my support and the container that holds and nourishes me.

A healthy marriage is one in which each party holds the other person's growth, success, and evolution as being as important as their own. It is difficult to describe the powerful impact of having her constant and unwavering belief in me and my vision to remind me of who I am and the value and importance of my work in times of self-doubt.

I married a woman who inspires me. Her commitment to her path, the depth and purity of her love for me, our child, herself, and the world is breathtaking. Her connection to her body, her emotions, and her trust in her intuition inspire me to understand and connect more deeply to these parts of myself.

As much as I thought that our timing was never right, in retrospect, I can now see that it didn't align to what I thought it *should* be and that it actually has the air of divine right timing. I now understand that I needed to go on an intense journey of exploration to understand myself, my masculinity, and my relationship to what it means to be a man. I had to deeply explore my own sexuality and to dive deep into my understanding of women and the feminine. I did so through a broad spectrum of women, each of whom added their own piece to the puzzle of my understanding through the things I got right and the things I got very wrong.

I can see now that if Elie and I had begun a romantic relationship at any point sooner than we did, it never would have worked. I still had so much of my shit to move through and many mistakes still to make.

I find a certain cosmic irony in the fact that I cultivated my Erotic Rockstar self, detail by detail, to become truly excellent at seducing women, yet nothing I learned in creating and becoming the Erotic Rockstar played a role in my relationship with Elie. We met before my Erotic Rockstar transformation, and she was in Japan during most of that phase. She stepped back into my life just as I was wrapping up that chapter. While I believe she still would have loved me, I don't think she would have chosen me in my Erotic Rockstar years to be her committed partner.

I look back on my Erotic Rockstar years as my epic hero's journey, during which I went beyond the edges of normal society and conventional thinking. I lived a wildly vibrant life that few would dare to and that most can't even fantasize about. I had an all-you-can-eat buffet of rich experiences, both light and dark, that has shaped me and given me a unique perspective on men, women, sex, and the world. As I let that mask fall away, I allowed the love of an empowered woman to change me. I slowly transitioned from being a polyamorous single man who picked up lovers wherever he went to being a committed husband and now father. That is a *massive* transformation in itself.

Elie has brought me stability, something that my life sorely lacked. She has brought me nourishment of my body, my health, and my heart. Within this container of our commitment and love, I have been able to build a successful business, which is rooted in my purpose and in creating a tangible impact in the world.

Early in our relationship, I started calling Elie "my gift from God." I felt as if I had leveled up. I felt as if I were being rewarded for a job well done and that I had learned the lessons I needed to learn in order to co-create a healthy, thriving relationship.

Committing to marriage is its own powerful transformational journey and is another step on my Evolved Masculine path. Sometimes I am challenged. Much of what I learned about how to be a man in the world doesn't apply now that I am married, especially now that I have a family. I liken it to playing a video game where you play a level again and again and get better and better, until you get so good that you can run through the level and hit a perfect score every time—but then you arrive at the next level, which has a completely new set of rules and objectives. All the skills you learned in the previous level have made you more skilled and more confident as you play in this new world—but it ultimately doesn't matter how good you were in that other world because this one is entirely different.

The word *sacrifice* has its roots in the Latin *sacrificim*, or "to make sacred." I sacrificed my Erotic Rockstar lifestyle in order to have the kind of family that I yearned for, and in so doing, I feel the sacredness of that family more fully. I am committed to being the best husband and father I can be, and once more, I don't always know what that looks like. There isn't an instruction manual, but I know now to seek out role models, to connect with other men who inspire me in the ways they model having a family. I know to surround myself with these men and to speak vulnerably about the challenges that arise for me, knowing that I do not need to do this all alone.

Every once in a while, I miss parts of my old lifestyle, but I look at what I have now, and it feels like a fucking miracle. There were many times during my Erotic Rockstar years that I thought that maybe it was just not in the cards for me to have that kind of lifelong love. Perhaps my lot in life was simply to have one torrid love affair after another. *Is that really so bad?* I would try to rationalize to myself, while all the while, in my heart of hearts, I yearned for it to not be true.

I believe that all of the times I loved and lost caused me to place an incredible value on the beautiful relationship I have with my wife. Elie went through a transformation of her own, from maiden to mother, with the birth of our first child. The woman I fell in love with was no more, as she became an entirely different version of herself as a gorgeous and devoted mom. Now I am learning to witness and love my wife through her own evolution.

While Kirsten catalyzed my Erotic Rockstar journey, Elie continually inspires me to deepen into my Evolved Masculine self. Each of my lovers taught me something about how to love a woman. However, in my marriage to Elie, I have learned whole new flavors of love. Love is sacrifice. My decisions aren't solely my own anymore. Every choice I make, I make in consideration of my wife and my family, as every choice I make affects them. Love is finding the delicate balance between sacrificing for my family and honoring my own need for self-nourishment. I learned that if I give to the point of depletion, my family is left with the weaker and darker parts of myself. Love is finding our way to forge a path forward while intertwining our lives *together*. The Evolved Masculine has learned to love.

54.
THE UNALOME

The entire Evolved Masculine path would not exist today if not for one badass Mr. Tung of Angel Art Tattoo Studio in Bangkok. Over the course of nine hours, this legendary artist inked a giant heart chakra piece upon my chest with the ancient symbol of the *unalome* positioned on six points of the tattoo. It was

the one part of my tattoo that I had nothing to do with. I didn't know a damn thing about the symbol, but now that it was suddenly part of a ten-by-ten-inch indelibly inked tattoo spread across my chest, I thought it might be a good idea to start looking into it.

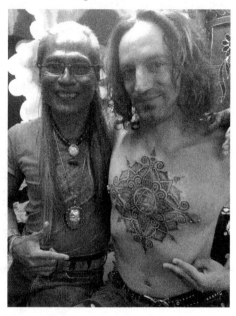

I discovered that the unalome is a Thai Buddhist symbol representing the path to enlightenment. The idea of a *path* has become deeply mean-ingful to me. It helps me make sense of my own lived experience. We live in a world that is obsessed with in-stant downloadable results, yet as I have gotten older, I have come to recognize that all that is truly meaningful is cultivated over time. This is the nature of a path.

When I was younger, I had the notion that life was supposed to be a progressive straight line: grow up, get good grades, go to a respected college, get married, settle down, have a family, work hard, retire, die.

I couldn't fit my life into this predetermined trajectory, and at points, I would see it as a failure on my part. On paper, my life does not make sense. I went way out of the box, actively breaking the chains of all the "shoulds" and "should nots" of societal conditioning, to discover my own distinct path. Only through learning to listen to and move from my inner truth was I able to discover my unique contribution to the world.

The symbol of the unalome that Mr. Tung etched onto my chest has become such a significant talisman to me that I built it into the logo for the Evolved Masculine. May it give you, too, a deeper understanding and acceptance of your own journey through life. The path is long and winding, but when traveled with increasing consciousness, it oscillates inward over time, winding tighter and tighter toward an essential truth of who you are. There may be times when you feel like you have failed or like you have gone "off path," yet as long as you maintain your commitment to your evolutionary growth, then there is no such thing as failure—it is *all* part of the path. *Fall down seven times, get up eight.* There were many times along the way at which I felt completely lost, yet looking back, I can now see the perfection in the strongly non-linear journey.

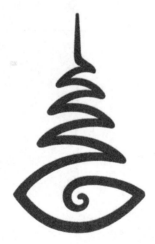

When I transformed myself from insecure, people-pleasing Greg into Destin Gerek, The Erotic Rockstar, I did so by killing off Greg. When I closed the chapter on the Erotic Rockstar and opened a new one with the Evolved Masculine, I did so by allowing the Erotic Rockstar to die. Now, through the writing of this book, my path pivots once more, as I am marking the transition into yet another evolution of self, one that includes the banished bravado of the

Erotic Rockstar, the still largely untapped potential of the Evolved Masculine, and the discipline and devotion summoned by being a father and a husband.

I am being pulled by a vision that I recognize will require a reclamation and integration of all the selves I have been before. The vision integrates all I have ever been with who I am now and who I continue to strive to become. The vision of this next chapter has been revealed to me, and this version of self will once again have to claw through the chrysalis in order to emerge strong enough to actively create this next potent chapter of my life.

In order for a man to live into his destiny, life becomes a necessary and sometimes ruthless repeating sequence of birth, death, and rebirth once more. If we cower in the face of our fear, we will miss the opportunity to create and leave behind the legacy of a lifetime.

The cave you fear to enter holds the treasure that you seek.

— Joseph Campbell

Some of the stories that I have shared with you were incredibly uncomfortable and edgy for me to write, let alone to publish for all the world to see. I chose to do so anyway, as I have learned that the greatest growth often comes from leaning into the places that feel terrifying. In the same way, I challenge you to lean in: lean in to the teachings here, and most importantly, lean in to your life.

I am acutely aware that some aspects of these teachings are provocative, controversial, and may not feel good to you in the moments of reading them. I do not expect for you to agree with everything I have written, and certainly not with every life choice I made along the way. I don't work that way, and I encourage you to challenge everything that is presented to you here. However, if there is a particular chapter or story that you find confronting, stay with it:

read it again, and wrestle with it. Bring it into the laboratory of your life, and test drive the fuck out of it.

There were many times over the years, during moments of great loss, rage, or confusion, when I raised my arms to the gods and questioned all that I was. I would then get the sense that I wasn't going through this for myself alone but that there was some way in which all of the incredible highs and devastating lows were in service to something greater than my individual self. Along the way, people have accused me of being grandiose in my thinking, but hell, I have used this belief to create an entire body of work and a successful company from it—*and thus made it so.*

I strongly recommend breaking out of any tendency you have to be a lone wolf and to instead build community with other men who are dedicated to walking a similar path of evolution and commitment to their potentiation. I have laid out a powerful path for you, but you are responsible for walking it. A potent key is resting in your hands that you can use to unlock an extraordinary life.

> I have also created a variety of resources for you, and will continue to create more. You can find them at:
>
> **http://EvolvedMasculine.com/book/resources**

I have laid my life on the line here for you because I know just how high the energetic costs were for me to learn the lessons I share here. If sharing these stories from my own life's journey makes your path a little bit easier, well, I will consider all the discomfort and pain of my struggles to have been worth it.

It is my hope that you can bypass a lot of the challenges and time that I went through in learning these lessons. Learn from my mistakes—and then go and make new and better mistakes of your own.

The path of the Evolved Masculine has four interlocking components, each of which requires some degree of mastery in order for you to create your life as a truly potent expression of who you are as a man.

If I could impress only one single principle from this book into the minds of all men (and all people, for that matter), it would be this: *you are a creator.* You carry within you the capacity to create any experience within this lifetime that you desire—and intentionally creating your life is worth every second of discomfort, every fleeting doubt, and every inconvenience. It will likely require hardcore dedication, as the undertow and program of complacency and mediocrity runs strong in our species. There will be many days where you will feel like you are caught in the crossfire between your current self and the iteration of self you know you can be.

Consciously creating *self* is one helluva commitment. It is not a path all men will choose to take, but those who do will one day know themselves as Godhead— and there is no more potent version of man that walks among us than the one who know himself as the creator he is.

The teachings I have shared with you have two primary thrusts: sex and creation. Your sex is deeply connected to who you are as a creator. Drawing from the front lines of my own lived experience, **Self as Creator** brings forward many pragmatic (with a hint of magic) tools and approaches to becoming the force of nature that is the truth of who you are . . . and who this world needs you to be.

Each of the **Lessons of the Evolved Masculine** were designed to powerfully re-veal intense experiences and aspects of my life that ultimately served as mega-watt "power-ups" in my evolution as a man. While your path will obviously look different in its details and circumstances, all men are—and will be—faced with significant tests and profound initiations. (Deep bow to women for their powerful capacity to call us out—and into—our best selves like nothing else on this planet.) As with the symbol of the unalome, the path of your life may not be the most direct, but there is a great intelligence operating beyond what things look like that is in direct service to your greatness.

Sexual Self-Mastery is the foundation for life mastery. Your capacity to know yourself as a free and powerful man is held within your sex, and specifically, in your relationship to mastering your sexual energy. Your sex is a potent force of energy, and once understood and embodied, it will radically your sense of self as a man. As you gain greater levels of sexual self-mastery, you will be able to experience and create greater degrees of pleasure. Even more than that, however, you will experience a surge in energy and a greater degree of freedom in your being. Claim this power, connect it with your heart, and use it with integrity and responsibility.

Lastly (although this is never last on the minds and in the hearts of men), **Understanding Women and** this mysteriously enchanting, sometimes dangerous thing called **the Feminine**: for a man to stand proudly and potently in his sense of self as a man requires that he make a deep commitment to a lifelong adventure of deepening and expanding his understanding of women and the feminine. Welcome her at your side, receive the gifts she has to offer, and ensure that her life is better for having met you.

Reading this book to completion indicates that you are committed to being the best man you can be. That said, reading a book isn't enough. To truly integrate this work and make it *part of you*, you must continue to hone your vision of your own Evolved Masculine self and commit each day to actively walking the path. The Evolved Masculine path, like all paths of self-mastery, does not have a set destination. Rather, it is a path you can dedicate your entire life to walking, and as each year passes and each new course correction is made, you can deepen into your self-mastery.

Thank you for investing the time and energy it took to read this book. While you may have picked it up for purely personal reasons, I would like to challenge you to take on a larger perspective. The entire reality of our planet is changing before our very eyes. I believe in you and know that you are needed. Your brothers need you. Women need you. The world needs you.

As the old saying goes, you can lead a horse to water, but you can't make him drink. My desire isn't simply to help you better reach your goals or have greater success with women. I want you to understand through embodied experience just how much capacity you have to create your life, and then to extend that ownership of yourself as a creator to take on the larger challenge and responsibility of helping to recreate the world around us. I believe that the women on this planet, the feminine as a force in this world, is calling forth a more Evolved Masculine, calling for us to show up and take on the responsibility of creating safety and space for the feminine in all her forms to flourish. We have within us the ability and responsibility to do just that. It isn't going to be easy, but nothing worth doing ever is.

If you are inspired with new possibility as a result of what you have read here, then I challenge you to rise up and become a man who inspires others.

The choice is yours. Will you choose to be the man the world needs and the one she craves? Your destiny is in your hands.

In service,

Destin Gerek

CRYSTALLIZE THE VISION OF YOUR EVOLVED MASCULINE ARCHETYPE: A GUIDED VISUALIZATION

The ideal way to get the most benefit from this guided visualization is to download it and listen to it on headphones with your eyes closed, really allowing yourself to be truly guided by my voice.

> Find it at:
> http://EvolvedMasculine.com/book/resources

If that is not possible, have a trusted friend guide you through the process by reading the following aloud while you sit, eyes closed, and allow yourself to be guided.

You can also record yourself reading the meditation out loud, and then play it back so that you are actually guiding yourself through this powerful process.

Now, let us begin . . .

When you are ready, close your eyes. Take this time to allow your breathing to really slow down and deepen. Settle in and find a place of quiet stillness within you. Bring your awareness to your sense of hearing, listening to the sounds in your environment, both loud and barely perceptible. Listen for the sound of your own breath. Bring your awareness to those sensations and feelings within your body as you slow down and deepen that breath even more. Allow your lungs to explore. What if these are the slowest breaths, the deepest breaths, that you have ever taken in your life? How slow would they be? How deep would they be?

From this place of breathing slowly and deeply, I want you to imagine . . . visualize . . . see in your mind's eye a path opening up before you. You notice that you immediately start walking down this path . . . or perhaps you have always been walking this path. One foot in front of the other, breath by breath.

Sometimes this path curves to the left, and you follow it to the left. Sometimes this path curves to the right; you follow it to the right. Sometimes the path slopes slightly downward, and the sun is shining, the wind is at your back; all seems right and easy in the world. Sometimes the path curves upward. As you walk, step by step, it gets steeper and steeper; maybe you even need to use your feet and hands to climb, making your way through, using every ounce of energy you have just to take the next step.

Bring your attention inward. Step by step, breath by breath.

Just when you are sure that you can't take another step, the path opens up onto a plateau. You climb onto this plateau and look out over a beautiful vista. What a gorgeous sight! As you stand there, just taking it in, you note that if you had given up at any point before—and there were times you wanted to—you would have missed all this. Here, you do not need to do anything. Simply allow yourself to soak in the beauty of your surroundings and this well-earned enjoyment.

After a while you realize that as beautiful as this is, you've got to keep moving. You know it is time to embark once again into the unknown and to continue on the path.

You see something ahead of you, out in the distance. What is this? A little glimmer of light of some kind. It appears to be a home, a dwelling of some sort. As soon as you see it, it is clear that you must head in its direction—or perhaps you have always been heading toward this home.

As you get closer, you start to make out the environment that this dwelling is in. Perhaps it is urban; perhaps it is rural. Or is it by the beach, or in the mountains? Perhaps it is surrounded by lakes, or desert, or trees. Just notice the environment that this home, this dwelling, is in.

All the while, slowly breathe in, and slowly breathe out, as you notice its details: what type of material is it made out of? How tall is it? What type of dwelling is it? Are there windows? How many? What are their shapes? Notice these little details, then make your way up to the front door.

As you stand outside of the front door, notice its color. What is unique or unusual about this door? Does it have a knocker or a handle? What is it like? Notice these little details.

As you raise your fist to knock, you pause, feeling that feeling in your belly—you know, that feeling — a mixture of nervousness and excitement—because you know who is on the other side of the door. Within this home lives . . . you—or a version of you, anyway. This version of you on the other side of the door has walked this path that you have walked, only he is a step, or maybe a few, ahead. This man on the other side of the door is your most fully integrated, activated, evolved version of yourself. This is the man who has claimed and owned and lived into his fully evolved masculine, who has integrated his healthy feminine, who has released any and all limiting beliefs, who has reached his fullest potential—this is the man on the other side of the door.

You knock. You hear footsteps coming toward you, and the door slowly opens. You see a figure standing there, bathed in light: powerful and radiant. What is the first thing that strikes you about this man before you? What do you notice about his energy? What does he look like? What clothes is he wearing? What are his shoes like? Is he even wearing shoes? What types of accessories is he wearing? Jewelry? Pendants? How does he style his hair? How is it similar to or different from how you appear today? What does his facial hair look like?

He greets you. Notice the words that he uses and the way in which he speaks them: notice his tone of voice, his pitch, his volume, and even the speed and cadence of his speech. After he greets you, he invites you in. Follow him into this dwelling. Notice the inside of the home. What does he surround himself with? What do you notice in his environment that he has consciously created for himself?

You stand before one another. You make eye contact with him, holding strong, powerful eye contact as you gaze into his left eye while he gazes into yours. This is an experiential exploration of the phrase "the eyes are the windows to the soul," as you recognize the paradox that you share the same soul. This man, this being, comes from the same essence that you do. Holding his gaze, you can feel an electricity, an energetic charge, moving between your eyes. You notice the qualities and attributes that are strongly within him. It is as if he has cultivated them to such a degree that he is generously sharing them with you. You feel as though by simply being in his presence and seeing him eye to eye, that with each of your inhalations you are able to breathe these resources, these attributes, deeper into your own being to whatever degree you have the capacity to hold in this moment . . . and perhaps it is more than you would have thought.

Now identify one attribute or quality that really strikes you about him. Hold the word for that attribute in your mind, then take a deep breath, as if you are breathing that quality in right now.

What other quality or attribute do you see in him at this time? What else strikes you about him? What inspires you? Hold that word, that attribute, in your mind, and once more, breathe it in with a deep inhale, and release with a long exhale. Keep these two attributes in your mind's eye, and remember the word you chose for each one.

Now a third quality or attribute about this man before you strikes you. What word or words do you use to describe it? Once more, breathe that in with a deep inhale, and release with a long exhale.

He says to you, "I've been waiting for you a long time. I'm sure you have questions for me."

You say, "Yes. For one, how did you get to be you?" or, "What can I do from where I am to start moving more intentionally in your direction?" Now ask that question in your own words, in your own way, and listen to his reply.

Once you have heard his answer, you have the opportunity to ask him anything, any question that is calling to you at this time. Formulate your question, and listen to his reply. Trust in the first thing that comes through.

Now find yourself with him in a new environment—maybe a more social environment—and notice how he is in the presence of other men; notice how other men respond to being in his presence and how he engages with them. Notice how women in his environment respond to him, both those whom he is overtly attracted to and those he is not. Notice how he interacts with them. Deep breath in. And deep breath out.

Now, come back before him, and see him before you eye to eye. As you do so this last time, shift your body into your most upright, confident, solid body posture that you can. Feel the shift in you as you stand there before him, eye to eye, matching and mirroring his way of being. As you hold this eye contact, he says to you, "This is a first meeting, not a last. Before we part ways, I want to leave you with something so that you know I am with you, and that you can call on me whenever it serves you."

He looks at you, eye to eye, as you gaze into him, and you can feel his piercing gaze; yet there is also a softness that allows you to gaze into him. Feel that power in your body, holding that strong posture, that breath within you. He reaches out and places his hand at the center of your chest. As he does so, you place your own hand on your chest, imagining and feeling his hand there.

He looks into your eyes and says something to you—I call it a power phrase. It is short, simple, and to the point, but it is exactly what you need to hear at this time. Feeling his hand on your chest, you see him eye to eye and hear him speak these words out loud to you. I invite you now to speak his words, this power phrase, out loud. See it. Go.

Breathe it in with a last deep inhale and exhale. See him eye to eye, feel his hand on your chest, and hear the phrase in his words. As you speak it out loud this time, mimic his way of speaking. Speak as he speaks. Speak this phrase once more—see it! Go.

Take a deep inhale and exhale. As you do so, feel yourself returning to this physical body. Feel the ground beneath you. Feel the breath in your body. Feel your butt touching the chair or ground below you. Tune in to hear the sounds in your environment. Give your fingers a little wiggle, your toes a little wiggle. As you are ready, allow your eyes to open, and come back.

Immediately following this guided visualization, pull out a notebook or open a document on your computer and write about what you just saw and experienced. The more detail you can write down, the more real it will become to you, and the easier it will be to access that connection again. This practice requires repetition to truly have the impact that it is meant to have.

I have included a short two-minute tune-up video on the book resources page to help you connect to your Evolved Masculine archetype as a regular practice.

http://EvolvedMasculine.com/book/resources

ACKNOWLEDGEMENTS

Writing this book required far more from me than I ever would have imagined. For years, people would ask where they could get my book. When I'd tell them that I hadn't written one yet, I'd universally get a strong nudge to please do so. Years continued to pass by and I'd watch one colleague after another publish their books, and still I resisted writing my own. *I know my work, but I don't know how to write a book,* I'd think to myself. *Besides, I'm more of a speaker than a writer.*

Finally, I relented. In retrospect, it would have been a very different book if I had written it back when people first started asking. I was still deep in my Erotic Rockstar chapter, and while I was already teaching for years by then, I was still very much *in* the experience. I can see things so much more clearly looking back on the whole journey.

It is impossible to name all those who helped me on my path to get here, so forgive the incompleteness...

I'd like to start by acknowledging Gillian Pothier without whom I can't imagine having successfully written a book that I would have been happy with. While her official title was developmental and content editrix, Gillian is a Jungian psychotherapist by training and truly helped me excavate my psyche and soul to draw out the right stories and express them coherently onto the page. She is an expert in masculine/feminine dynamics in her own right and would challenge me on my ideas until they were honed more precisely and expressed in the best way possible. She pushed, poked, and prodded me, unafraid to make me uncomfortable so long as it would result in better writing. I don't know what I expected when I brought Gillian on to support me in this book, however whatever it was, she exceeded all expectations.

I must acknowledge Jaiya, the first person that I knew personally to write a best-selling book. In the thirteen years that I've known her, Jaiya has always been a source of inspiration for me, showing me what is possible when you are truly dedicated to your purpose. Thank you Jaiya for being a friend.

Thank you Joseph Kramer for being an early mentor, for seeing me, believing in me, and helping me lay a foundation of both erotic embodiment and integrity that has informed my path ever since.

Thank you Jonathan and Heike Hudson for allowing Gillian and I to spend days and long nights in your home writing tirelessly while you encouraged me all the while.

Thank you Jim House for helping me map out an initial outline of the content that I wanted to bring forward.

Thank you to the early supporters and believers in my work: Rhett Bise, Steven 'Open Heart' Vymola, Larry Davidson, Andrew Goad, Ryan Junee, Rion Kati, Joe Mattia, Bertram Meyer, Michael Author, Dave McDermott, and so many others.

Thank you to my advanced readers for taking the time to read the book in its unfinished form and provide feedback that allowed me to improve it for others: Eric Clopper, Chace Spillman, Akira Chan, Zev Daniels, and Niraj Mehta.

Thank you to Rich Litvin for helping me see how much more I was capable of. *Perfect vulnerability is perfect protection.* Well then I should be ok, because damn did I get vulnerable.

Thank you Martha Bullen for all of your support in the publishing process.

Thank you mom for teaching me to be myself and not worry about what other people think of me. Thank you dad for instilling in me 'if you set your mind to it, you can do anything.' These two teachings together have proven to be a powerful combination.

To each of the incredible women who have touched my life (some named and many others who were not): You inspired me. You challenged me. And the two together have made me a better man. Thank you…

And of course, most of all, I must thank Elie for being the most incredible wifey ever. Thank you for putting up with the many, many deadline extensions, and all the ways that you took on more in order to make sure that I had the time and focus that I needed to write. I don't think it's a coincidence that I didn't finally write this book until I was married to you. I have never felt so supported in my hopes and dreams, my well-being and my happiness, as I feel with you. I know that I wasn't as present with the family as I would have liked to have been while writing this book. I also know that I am not the easiest husband in the world, but I am committed to being an ever better man, as you deserve nothing less.

My daughter Inanna, as you grow, may the men that you meet strive to understand you, protect you, and serve you on your own personal and spiritual journey. May the world be a better and safer place for you to grow up in as a result of my efforts here and in all that I do. Thank you for coming into my life and inspiring me in a whole new way.

CONNECT:

I'd love to hear how this book has impacted you!

Find me on Social Media:

f fb.com/destingerek

⊡ @EvolvedMasculine

🐦 @DestinGerek

▶ youtube.com/destingerek

Share your stories with the hashtag #EvolvedMasculine

The Evolved Masculine podcast
Available on your favorite podcast platform

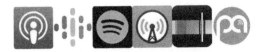

Step into YOUR Evolved Masculine Power!

If you are ready to take the ideas that you've just read about in this book and apply them more deeply to bring about radical transformation in your own life, then join me for this **FREE 60-minute** webinar training.

http://EvolvedMasculinePower.com

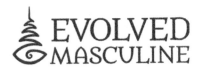

ABOUT THE AUTHOR

Destin Gerek is an internationally recognized leading voice in masculinity, sexuality, and personal empowerment. Destin is founder and CEO of The Evolved Masculine, a pioneering coaching and training company for men and host of the podcast, *"The Evolved Masculine: Redefining Sex, Power, & Success"*. His innovative lens is the result of more than 20 years of academic rigor and direct study — including 7 formative years traveling the world living and teaching as his provocative alter ego, *'The Erotic Rockstar'*. Destin has taken the most potent aspects of his bold life experimentation and integrated it into his iconic body of work, directly supporting thousands of men to have better sex, deeper connections to their masculine power, women, and themselves.